THE BUILD IT

BLUEPRINT

BUILD MUSCLE. BUILD STAMINA. BUILD STRENGTH.

By

DOUG BENNETT

Top American Trainer

BUILD IT is guaranteed the most complete meal-by-meal, day-by-day training program in the fitness market for guys over 30. It's going to show you how to get maximum results whether you're trying to get fighting fit, pack on muscle or just get into top shape without living in the gym!

Are you ready to pack on muscle, build strength, increase stamina, boost testosterone and feel healthy without living like a body builder?

Are You 30 to 50 years old and fall into one of the 4 categories?
1. The Busy Executive who needs a guaranteed get super fit plan to that is doable in between both work and family?
2. The Single Guy who wants to pack on muscle and get the look the ladies are attracted too?
3. The Ex-Athlete who was a star high school or college athlete who hates the gym, but wants to get into top shape to play the sport he once loved or simply wants to get into fighting shape?
4. The Guy who's a combination of all 3 plus needs to lose belly fat and once to transform his fat ass?

Then this book is for you. BUILD IT brings your goals to reality.

You're going to get everything you need to get fit fast, feel healthy, lose belly fat, pack on muscle, boost testosterone and build confidence.

This is not for bodybuilders. This is for guys who have a real life who don't want to live in the gym like an 18 year old who checks out his biceps, eats boiled carcass and protein bars.

This book gives you diet options and workouts that will fit into your busy life and give you the results you desire. This isn't about eating grass and drinking green drinks. Nor is it about working out with a rubber band and telling you that you'll look like a fitness model. The diets and workouts are the real deal!

MESSAGE FROM DOUG BENNETT

"If you're going to just read this book without taking action (following the meal plans and most importantly, using the workouts) then spare me a review and don't buy this book. This is only for those who want to change the way they look and feel. This is an action taking book and not for those who think reading scientific shit is going to get them in shape. If you want all the science go take a fucking college class. You've got to put in some intense effort to maximize results in less time. I've taken out all the fluff and given just the stuff that works."

Doug Bennett

One more thing:

Yes, this book will allow you to pack on muscle, lose belly fat increase testosterone and build confidence without eating just salad and boiled chicken. Yet, you must use the workouts and give 100% effort.

None of these workouts in this book have ever been seen. It's not about just putting 10 of this and 10 of that together just to fill pages No punching the air, no eating Lean cuisine, no performing tricep bench on a chair nor jumping around to a DVD in your underwear.

Doug Bennett, one of Americas Top Trainers, has helped professional athletes, Olympic wrestlers and thousands of guys who just want to look and feel their best.

Now, he's decided to share some of his knowledge on paper for less than a six pack. You'll save thousands of dollars and wasted hours on trying to figure out what works by downloading The Build Your Body Blueprint today!

All intellectual property created by Douglas Bennett including

The Build It and/or doug Bennett, author, writes an exact diet and workout system that can get you into your best shape ever. However, you must use it to get your desired results. Always, consult a qualified medical professional before starting this or any other diet and fitness program. You are assuming all risk and liability by reading and using any of the material written in the Build It and/or created by Douglas Bennett. Always stop if you feel discomfort and seek medical help immediately.

TABLE OF CONTENTS

Your busy Guide blueprint to a Buff and Fit body..

Let me start out by thanking you for taking the time and a

Slither of belief that this book will actually help you get fit and muscular even if you have failed before or think you don't have the time to work out.

I'm hoping by the end of this book you will eliminate all chemicals and bad stuff from your diet and change the way you work out forever. Yes, I guarantee once you use my programs you'll see what a pro-level training is like. I won't even make you jump up holding your crotch, perform squats on a chair or anything like that crap. All these workouts are original and aren't like 99% of the copy cat training programs in the fitness market.

Let's face it, you need a program that gives you fastest results possible while letting you focus on the daily grind: a job, bills, kids, and everyday time sucking activities.

Yet, before you go any further. I'm telling you now.

This is not a body-building program.

I repeat:

You will not be a meat-head from this plan. This plan is for those guys who want to live a healthy lifestyle, get super fit and be able to kick some ass if need be.

I'm going to show you everything a guy from 30-50 years old needs to pack on muscle, lose fat, live healthy, drop pounds and all the shit that goes with it.

ABOUT ME

So, you're probably saying "who is this guy"? "What does he know?" "I've heard all this shit before! Well, I'm not a "so-called" guru who was a fat, dumpy pussy (and still is) who has eaten fast food his whole life and all of the sudden has started to eat sub rolls and salads to lose weight or is a 20 year old trainer who lifts in the gym 2 hours a day and thinks he's tough because he can't lift his arms.

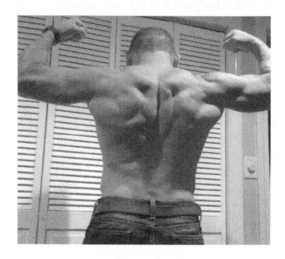

My dedication to intense training and eating right helped me land a spot on the Clemson University Wrestling Team, a top ranked Division 1A wrestling college at the time. Unfortunately, due to a major infection and a knee injury I was sidelined and was forced to only lift. Most guys thought I was on steroids at the time, but honestly I just knew what to do and how to put on mass. Guys noticed and I was writing programs for all the Top Athletes for Clemson back in the late eighties.

Fast Forward many years, I graduated with a B.S. in science/nutrition, own a very successful training center and have personally trained thousands of clients from Pro-Athletes, Olympic Wrestlers, UFC athletes, Division 1A College Teams, CEOS, just to name a few.

As a father of 2 boys at 47 years old. I train clients 60 to 70 hours a week, so believe me I know how hard it is to fit a workout into your day. So, you're not alone. Follow this book and you'll see how to get fit fast.

So, to summarize all this crap, I've been a trainer for 27 years and know what works for guys of all levels of training. I promise once you try my training method, you'll see what makes me different and why

I get paid $125- $250 for just one private 30 minute training session.

WHAT'S YOUR GOAL?

I've designed this book so you can select which guy best fits your lifestyle and goal. Obviously, if you're 30 years old you'll have different goals then a guy who's 50 years old. So, I've created a different program for 3 different guys based upon their goal.

Guy 1 is the Business Guy: he's motivated to look and feel good. He wants to look fit and muscular but not like a body builder. He's always on the go and travels a lot. So, he needs a diet that incorporates eating out and entertaining. His workouts need to be fast, effective and versatile (gym, travel and home).

Guy 2 is the Single Guy: he's got more time to workout (30-90 minutes a day). He wants to pack on muscle and lose fat so he can pick up the ladies. He's willing to eat a more bland diet just to look good.

Guy 3 is the Sports Guy: he was a former athlete who wants to get back into his favorites sport (basketball, hockey, tennis, etc.). He wants to drop pounds, build strength, increase stamina, feel healthy and look good again. He's got a busy schedule along with a family.

One thing they all have in common:
They don't want to live in a gym or look like a meat head.

So, step 1:
Pick the guy who most sounds like you.

LETS GO OVER THE BORING SHIT

Look, I'm not going to fill up these pages with a bunch of bullshit. I'm going to get right to the point and tell you exactly what you need to know and do.

Nothing bothers me more than reading a plethora (Big sat word) of material that can be said in few words. Look, I'm not an English major, so pardon me for my bad English, but I will help kick your ass into shape. Please, if you're just going to read this book and not use the workouts. Don't review it. Return it. Go eat a pizza and go back to your aerobics class.

NUTRITION YOU NEED TO KNOW

First, <u>you don't need</u> to know the cell properties or the chemical compositions of all the basic food groups. However, you should learn some basic nutrition concepts in order to get and stay fit. These nutrition basics should be put into your daily habits.

Man Rule #1

**Eat lean and clean protein with each meal
(No nitrates, free range and minimally processed, if at all)**

To build the most muscle, you should use high protein sources like lean meats, eggs, etc. which get broken immediately into amino acids that are used by repairing and growing muscle cells.

Hence, *not all protein sources are created equal.* That's why you should eat the best protein sources throughout the day.

Here's how to get a rough idea of how much protein you should take in a day:

1. Divide your weight in half and multiply it by 1.5 grams if you weigh less than 175 lbs. if you're bigger than 175 lbs. than multiply your half weight by 2 grams.

Example: you start out at a mere 100lbs. divide by 2 = 50lbs x 1.5 = 75 grams protein.

2. Now, divide that by 3-6 meals and your good to go.

SHORT-CUT: Make it simple. Try to eat protein sources, 4-6 x day. If you can only get your protein portions in only 3 meals, no big deal. Try to increase the amount of protein in each of those 3 meals. Don't fret about getting your perfect amount of amino acids in each meal as you're not trying to look like a body building freak. Believe me, being a body builder is not going to make you tough.

PROTEIN POWER TIPS

- ✓ Protein powder in smoothies coupled with glutamine powder after each weight training session is optimal for recovery and muscle development.
- ✓ Slow eating and extra chewing helps with protein absorption.
- ✓ Always drink extra water with each protein meal.
- ✓ Try to eat salad and some fibrous fruit between or with a protein meal. Both aid in digestion.
- ✓ Please don't believe pork is the other white meat. Ham, pork, sausage and processed hot dogs are way off the radar. Yeah, you're a guy but you don't' want to be a lard ass either. If you think like a Jew (I'm half Jewish) you'll make the right choices, ha…
- ✓ Vegetarians should add the following supplements to their diet: iron, magnesium and branched chain amino acids.
- ✓ Keep raw nuts in the fat section. Yes they contain protein but to get lean and fit we are going to treat them as a good fat.
- ✓ Cholesterol issues? Before you just eat chicken and fish…think again. Check with your doctor.

Should you divide By 6 meals?

No, that's for the meat heads. Hopefully, you're working on financial success and you're concerned about making money. You'll be fine if you eat 3 meals and 3 lean snacks. If you're retired,

And can actually eat 5-6 meals a day, then you're lucky. *If you eat every other hour you'll be certain to absorb more than enough of those little branched chain aminos.*

Face it, if you want a flatter stomach and some quality muscle development, then do you think you should be mowing corn puffs, bagel chips and candy bars? Of course not. Stick to a diet that's going to give you flat abs: steak, chicken, eggs and fish. *The more you incorporate lean protein into your diet, the less hungry you'll be and your craving for sugar will diminish.*

You might as well eat the best protein you can. Below, I've given you the best sources of protein to choose from.

Six Pack Protein Choices

EGG Whites: egg Whites and more egg Whites. Like eggs? Then don't be scared to eat 1-2 whole eggs. Egg yolks have hidden vitamins, minerals and other good stuff.

You're best to mix 1 whole egg to 2-3 egg whites. Try to buy free range eggs. Why try to eat more egg whites rather than eating all eggs. Yes, yolks are ok but they do contain fat. Fat is ok but that doesn't mean you should mow it down. If you want to eat 2 hardboiled eggs, then fuck it, no big deal. You're going to be a workout machine when you use this book.

Meat: top sirloin, flank, top round steak, buffalo, Turkey, chicken, turkey bacon, lean (93%-98%) ground beef/ turkey/ chicken/bison

Vegetarian: edamame, beans, seeds, lentils, raw nuts, brown rice, wheat berry, organic tofu, quinoa, tempeh.
   *lentils are your best choice mixed with wheat berry and raw nuts.

Dairy: cottage cheese, Greek yogurt (2%-5%), Eggs (egg whites)

*Make sure you buy organic cottage cheese as the rest of them are packed with preservatives. If you're on a low salt diet then keep away from these foods.

Fish: white fish, salmon, crab, tuna, salmon, scallops, shrimp

Protein Powders: hemp, whey, brown rice, egg, pea, quinoa
*Make sure you're buying an organic and natural protein powder without additives, soy and artificial flavors.

MY TOP PICKS:

Build MASS: lean beef, and broiled chicken on the bone, dark meat and Grass Fed Whey Protein

Get LEAN: Egg Whites, Hemp Protein, Fish, Lentils

Foods That Suck For a Protein Source:
- Pork
- Soy products
- Bacon
- Sausage
- Organ Meats
- Protein Bars, Protein Processed Foods i.e. cereal, ice cream

Golden Rule #1:

Eat lean, free range (whenever possible) protein sources throughout the day (6-8x to build mass / 4-5x to get lean). Don't eat hot dogs, ham, pork and pork sausages. Don't be a lard ass.

Think about the inside of your body and not just how you look. It's like the body builder who looks ripped but inside his liver is failing and his heart is ready to implode from all the steroids.

More Protein Shit You Need To Know

If you're not lifting weights or training hard then forget about supplements or eating extra protein. Extra protein, supplements and amino acids will do shit other then make you shit more.

Soy protein is mostly over processed. Stay away from foods that are soy protein fortified. i could cite lots of research that backs this up but take it for what it's worth. If you're a soy lover than stick to organic tempeh and organic tofu.

Protein bars are not a good source of protein. They suck. You're better off eating a green apple and some raw almonds. You can buy some dried buffalo much like a beef jerky (see brand recommendations). You don't have to worry that much that you can't wait for a meal. Simply shaking your powder with coconut water or low-fat milk is an option if you want to get another protein meal while on the go. Oh yea, don't forget about keeping hardboiled eggs on hand.

Read all labels. Foods that say "a good protein source" on the front package most likely are no good. Unless it's clean protein from the good protein foods then it's probably not good protein. Example: protein ice cream.

Protein Questions Answered:

Can I eat steak every day?
Hmm. I wouldn't. If you do make sure it's one of the lean sources and break it up throughout the day. If you're 200 pounds then eating 16 ounces of steak is no big deal. However, if you're 150 pounds and eating 16 ounces of steak 2x/day then you may have a problem.

Hey, if you don't believe me, then eat steak 1-2/day for a week. Then, void beef the next week and see how you feel. Animal protein is great for muscle building, but remember that you have arteries. Arteries love to attract plaque caused by excessive fat, and protein.

So, I personally would recommend that you limit beef to 2-3x a week and choose lean, free-range cuts as much as possible.

Is Peanut Butter a Good Source Of Protein?

Unfortunately, you'll need to consume too many unnecessary calories from peanut butter to get the protein needed to build quality muscle. You could eat a lot more chicken for the same amount of calories and get a lot more protein to build muscle. Raw Nuts are great to satisfy hunger pains and incorporate good fats into your diet.

How Can I Naturally Absorb More Amino Acids?

1. Drink lots of water.
2. Eat pineapple and/or drink *pineapple juice which is high in bromelain* (protein enzyme).
3. Purchase a protease enzyme at your local health food store.
4. Train with heavy weights and intensity
5. Choose only Clean Protein Sources i.e. fish and not bars

Is It True If I Eat More Protein the More Muscle I'll Develop?

Yes, and no. Your body will only process a limited amount of protein in every meal. You can figure all that out as you lift. The great thing about our bodies is that it responds to your diet and workouts. The *more intense you train, the more protein you should consume for muscle repair and growth. Overall, you need to consume protein to get more amino acids to build muscle.* They don't just make themselves from food sources such as sugar.

What's the best protein powder to buy?

I personally think hemp protein is a superior protein for health, digestion and will help you build muscle. Yes, better than whey protein.

Short-Cut:
If you weigh 175 lbs. or less, then eat 1/2 a fistful of protein (approx. 3-4 ounces each meal, 3-6 meals a day).

If you're between 17lbs and 240 lbs.

Then consume ¾ of a fistful of protein (approximately 4-6 ounces per meal, 3-6 meals a day).

If you're over 240lbs. (greater than 24% body fat), then revert back to childhood and consume the same protein intake as your 150 lb. buddy.

Make sure you drink more than enough water, daily. Drinking water with each and every meal is crucial for protein digestion.

Experiment with your protein intake. You'll actually begin to get in tune with your body the more fit you get.

Should I eat only protein?
NO!!!! Remember when everyone was just eating a high protein diet? Guys didn't care what they ate as long as it said protein. They were eating foods like: bacon, ham, pork, pork rinds, sausage, peanuts just to name a few.

Leading to what? Well, it led to guys hobbling down the street with gout, heart disease and all kinds of digestive problems.

Eat a balanced diet (like grandma said). Eat lean protein, six pack carbs, fruits, veggies and good fats. This diet will lead to more energy, better sex (she's happier), confidence and a cleaner body.

Can I Build Muscle On a Vegetarian Diet?
Yes. Actually, if you cut out all meat from your diet and eat strictly *a diet that balances legumes, hemp protein, tempeh (organic), lentil and brown rice, raw nuts, seeds and a complete amino acid based*

supplement, then you'll actually feel great! One problem. You may increase your energy so much you may buzz around like a rabbit in heat.

I Don't Know What To Eat for Breakfast That's High In Protein?

Breakfast Ideas Higher In Protein:
- Free Range chicken or turkey sausage mixed with roasted sweet potato and turnips
- English muffin egg sandwiches:
- Bowl of hemp seeds, chia seeds, almonds and steel cut oats.
- Organic Steak, egg and cheese.
- Ground bison with chopped tomato and egg
- Natural Turkey Bacon, egg whites and cheese.
- Natural Turkey or Chicken sausage, egg whites and cheese.
- Free Range Chicken, egg and cheese omelet.
- Natural turkey bacon, guacamole and egg whites.
- Low-fat cottage cheese, dates and nuts
- Lean Steak and eggs
- Hard-boiled egg, Organic Greek Yogurt and Kind bar
- Egg White Omelets or Scrambled Egg Whites
- Salmon spread on Lundberg Brown Rice Cakes
- Protein Smoothies (2-3 scoops powder: casein, whey and/or hemp)
- Organic apple with **raw butter Protein spread (see recipe)**
- Ezekiel Toast with raw nut (cashew or almond butter)
- Protein Raw Butter (see recipe below) spread on a **Lundberg** Brown Rice Cake.

Protein Raw Butter Recipe
Take your favorite raw butter (almond or cashew butter) and place the entire jar in blender. Add 1 cup water, 8 scoops natural vanilla or chocolate whey protein powder. Blend until smooth.

MAN MOMENT: Try a vegetarian diet for 1 week. Just 1 week. Test your will power and see how you feel. If you're are saying, "No way!" then just eat free range chicken and fresh fish for protein in your diet.

Sometimes, it's great to eat a vegetarian diet for 1-2 days every month to kick your metabolism up and flush out your body. I'll give you a sample of a vegetarian diet later in the book.

Man Rule #2

Complex Carbs are as important as lean protein to building a strong and muscular body

---

Let's make this simple as possible. To lose weight fast you really should limit your sugar intake. Think of sugar as your bodies enemy.

Yet don't fall for the trend that, "all sugar is bad for you!" if that was the case, then your brain wouldn't be effectively working. All your cells need sugar to work. That goes for muscle cells especially. Carbs are needed for your heavy lifts. You don't need a lot but you need some or you'll be weak, tired and frustrated.

NOTE: if you don't have the sugars available in the form of glycogen stored from complex carbs. Your body will naturally break down amino acids needed for muscle development and convert them into sugars.

Plus, unless you have to lose 20 lbs. plus. Don't worry about eating foods with a little sugar. That's you you're going to lift like a mad man. Don't be a fucking girly man. No lady wants to be with a guy who's all ripped up. Well, 99% of them anyhow and the ones that do usually have so much muscle they should have a dick.

Your Muscle Cells need stored sugars (glycogen) for fast-acting activities (anaerobic): punching, sprinting, skating, fast jump rope etc.; and mid-range endurance activities (aerobic): jogging, biking, etc....

Carb Power Tips

- ✓ If you're trying to drop 10 pounds: Complex carbs should make up 20-30% of your first and second meal, 5 % for third meal.
- ✓ If you're trying to keep your six pack. Complex carbs should make up 30-40% of your first meal, 30-50% of your second meal, and 10% for third meal.
- ✓ If you're running less than 6-8 miles than you really don't need to eat carbs before exercising.
- ✓ Eat a complex carb source within hour after exercising. Especially lifting.
- ✓ Eat high fibrous fruits after an intense training session: oranges, pears, green apple, berries, melon, grapefruit
- ✓ A sports drink with fructose or dextrose immediately after an intense WEIGHT TRAINING SESSION does help with glycogen (energy) replenishment.

Do you think only smoking a pack of cigarettes is the only thing that will give you a heart attack? Think again. White sugar and better yet, white flour is just as bad.

A diet made up of mostly sugar, (note: I said mostly) no matter where the sugars come from, can lead to obesity, diabetes type 2 and all kinds of other health issues. Plus, it gives you that nice fat gut that makes you sound like a beached whale flapping against the wet sand while you're on top of your girlfriend.

Foods to Eliminate From Your Diet (if you want good results and live healthy):

Baked Goods, Soda, Diet Soda, Artificial Sugars, Molasses, Honey, Corn Syrup, White Rice, All flour, 99% Cereals, Protein Bars, Corn Bread, Pastries, Candy, White Rice Cakes, Bread, Apple Juice, Processed Foods, Dressings, Tortilla Chips and so on.

Golden Rule # 2:

Read the ingredients before you eat or buy it. Don't believe the marketing. Look for dextrose, artificial sweeteners, glycols, and all the shit.

Carbs Best For Your Body:

Short Grain Brown rice, Beans, Barley, Yams, Potato, Bulgur Wheat, Wheat Berry, Quinoa, Carrots, Whole Oats, Wild Rice, Brown Rice Cakes and Root Veggies.

Weight Loss Tip:

Try to stick to yams, lentils, root veggies and turnips as a snack or lunch if you're trying to lose those last stubborn pounds.

Power Carb Tips:

✓ Always select natural, whole foods (all natural and unprocessed ingredients). Once you take out all processed foods from your diet, you'll find yourself craving less sugars.

✓ Eat small, frequent portions of good carbs. Your body after a week or two will give you an indication of what portions are best (hence, you'll have more energy, less bloat and your muscles will feel tighter)

✓ Eat a complex carb immediately after a strenuous training session

✓ Eat a handful of organic nuts in place of a sugar craving. Throw some organic dried fruit in there too.

- ✓ Drink 8 ounces of organic orange juice with pulp in the morning. The acidity and sweetness seems to satisfy sugar cravings
- ✓ Increase your fiber intake. Fiber will diminish the sugar spike.
- ✓ Beans are more of a carb source and high in fiber.

CARBOHYDRATE QUESTIONS ANSWERED:

Can I eat foods made of wheat flour?

Flour is already refined down and gets broken down into sugar once inside the body. So, no matter what flour you're eating. If you eat too much, your body will handle it as excess calories which will be stored as glycogen or fat. Most likely, fat and you'll hold water around the belly.

So, unless you want to eat pasta or a piece of pizza once in a while. Stay away from all flour. If you do eat products made with flour, it the higher fiber source like wheat or brown rice flour. **Remember, if you're lifting heavy and intense, you'll utilize the perfect portion of pasta or white rice.**

Oh you like cookies? Grow up. Make or buy some snacks that are just rolled oats, whole grains with stuff you like in them (nuts, dried fruit, etc.)

Dinner Tip: if you can't keep your face from devouring 3 to 5 of those dinner rolls, simply tell your waiter to skip the rolls and bring a healthier appetizer. Obviously, salad is your best bet or tuna is my favorite.

Lunch Tip: you're at a sub shop and you really want a sandwich. What bread do you use? Sub roll, Pita, Lettuce or Wrap? Choose the Lettuce first and pita second! Skip the bread all together if possible. Choose the crappy salad. There are so many healthier options to choose from. Forget going to your local deli or pizza joint.

Why Do I Lose Weight Fast When I Cut Out Carbs?

Carbs in general attract water molecules more than proteins and fats. So, when you cut carbs out of your diet you initially lose water weight.

You can drop 5-10lbs. quickly by just cutting out flour and sugar within 1 to 3 weeks. *White flour, gluten and sugar will hinder your body from looking its best.*

Plus, carbs in general are easy to gobble down without realizing you just had eaten 2 meals worth of calories.

Is eating Carbs One Day and not the Next Good?

Carb loading or Carb Cycling is an old trick of storing glycogen (stored sugar) for competition. Simply, eat the carbs that are good for you every day and train like a mad-man. You'll enjoy eating, and you'll spend less time thinking about guys in thongs posing up on stage..

What If I Want To Cut Out Carbs Completely?

Sure. Fuck it. Suffer. Just don't cut fruit, water and veggies from your diet. May be tough to live with your family.

What about Alcohol?

It's a simple fact that alcohol contains lots of non-nutritional calories that can pack on pounds quickly, lower testosterone, deplete your body from nutrients, dehydrate your muscles and the list goes on.

I personally don't drink but I understand I'm an anomaly. A drink once or twice a week won't kill you. You can be the judge of how you feel. Believe me, once you start eating clean and you mess up by eating something that's unhealthy. You 'll get a food hangover just as bad as if you drank the night before (headache, bloat, tired, sluggish and so on).

Is Bread Really Bad For You?

Most breads are made of fillers, additives, sugars, gluten and refined flours.

Just because a package says, "wheat" doesn't mean shit. Most likely it's just masked white bread with brown food coloring.

Bread should have at least 3 grams of fiber per slice. Try to limit your bread intake to 3-4 meals per week. For the last 21 years my only choice of bread has been Ezekiel.

Until recently, fitness trainers are just beginning to learn about it. The Food For Life Brand breads taste great and have a flourless variety. I make sandwiches with toasted Ezekiel English Muffins or Engine 21 hamburger rolls (egg, tuna, turkey, shaved steak, ground meat and chicken).

Can I eat Pizza?

Is your goal to have a six pack? If yes, skip the pizza. If no, then limit to 1-2 slices and eat only from naturally made ingredients. Don't expect to be and look your best if you eat pizza every day. Yet, don't be worried about eating it once a week. Make sure to lift heavy the next day.

I need to gain muscle and weight?

To get full, well-rounded muscle development, glucose refueling is important for muscle recovery after weight training. Complex carbs (brown rice, quinoa, oats) and a mix of fruit (berries, watermelon and mango are great after a heavy lift). To help gain weight, eat extra complex carbs with every meal. Make sure to lift heavy with intensity.

A post-workout meal can be a 3:1 or 4:1 carbohydrate to protein ratio. An example of a post workout (weight training) meal can be any of the following: baked potato with organic cottage cheese and pineapple, chicken breast with a bowl of brown rice, mango and corn/

black bean, brown rice and organic ground turkey, protein drink with fruit, steak and sweet potato or wild rice.

Should I use Artificial Sweeteners?

Never use any artificial sweeteners. You're better off using raw cane sugar, stevia, agave, honey, or 100 % maple syrup. Artificial sugars can trick your brain to store fat. Digestion happens at the tongue. Your mind is triggered by sweetness and tells your hormones in your body to act a certain way to digest foods.

Golden Rule #3:

Eat complex carbs for fuel and to build a great body.

Man Rule #4

**Eat Good Fat For Good Health and Testosterone.
Eat lots of Bad Fat and You'll Be a Fat Shit.**

Fats in the form of polyunsaturated and monounsaturated fatty acids are beneficial to cardiovascular health, immunity, vitamin absorption, metabolic processes, energy, ligament stability testosterone and losing weight.

Although good fats are healthy. That doesn't mean you can just eat them with no consequence. There are 9 calories/gram so the calories can add up quickly.

STAR THIS SHIT:

Even though good fats are good for your health. Don't consume good fats 4-6 x day, _if you need to lose 15 pounds or greater._ This means not adding avocado, hummus, oil and other fats to your diet 3-6x day. Eating seeds and a few nuts are ok. Yet, don't eat a high fat diet intake till you hit your goal weight.

To cook, use broths, organic non-stick sprays or water.

Power Fat Tips For Better Health

- ✓ Add a good fat to your salads and veggies (example: extra virgin olive oil, "Earth balance" butter spread.
- ✓ Spectrum brand oils are great. Make sure you cook only with high heat cooking oils with heat. Almond, peanut, avocado oil and Sunflower oil.
- ✓ Omega 3 fatty acids are a good source of fat and are found in many fish (salmon and swordfish).
- ✓ If you're trying to pack on a little weight then add avocado and some raw nut 3 times a day to your diet.

Fats That Make You Fat and Unhealthy:

Animal Fat, Hydrogenated Fat, Artificial Butters, Palm Oil, Dairy Fat, Cotton Seed Oil, Frying Oils, Trans Fatty Acids, Tropical Oils,

Margarine, Processed Butter

Good for Your Body Fats (eat sparingly if trying to lose weight)

Cod Liver Oil, Raw Nuts, Salmon, Sardines, Extra Virgin Olive oil, Coconut oil (organic), Grape Seed Oil (organic), Almond Oils (organic), Seeds (chia, sunflower, hemp, and flax), Avocado

Man Rule #5

Consume Fresh Spring Water throughout the Day

Your body needs lots of water. Drink water, water and more of the shit. Water keeps you from cramping, increase your metabolism (energy) and is crucial to deliver important nutrients to your muscles. If you start to feel sluggish or hungry, drink water and see if that takes care of the problem. I could go on and on about the benefits but I won't. Just drink it.

- ✓ Water + muscle = Better metabolism
- ✓ healthy skin & muscle Tone = healthy Water intake
- ✓ sweat = double Water consumption
- ✓ Pee is clear = good
- ✓ Wake Up = drink Water
- ✓ heavy Water Loss = Take a multiple Vitamin and multimineral complex

Power Water Tip

Drink fresh spring water 5-6 x per day at least. Start Off your morning with water and a squeeze of a fresh lemon.

Man Rule #6

Fiber helps stabilize blood sugar and a healthy digestive system

Insoluble fibers (bran) are not digestible in the small intestine and soluble fibers (legumes) are digestible. Soluble fibers are the best form of fiber for lowering your cholesterol and for slowing glucose absorption in the small intestine.

Below are some quick tips to increase your daily fiber intake:

- ✓ Add 1-2 tbsp.: oat bran or wheat germ to your smoothie, oatmeal or salad.
- ✓ Eat an apple a day
- ✓ Add berries and legumes to your salad
- ✓ Handful of organic trail mix with almonds, seeds and raisins
- ✓ Eat 1-2 mixed green salads per day
- ✓ Eat 1-2 biscuits of Barbara's Shredded Wheat every day as a snack or breakfast.

Foods Higher In Fiber:

Apples, Corn, Dried Prunes, Broccoli, Berries, Oats, Flax, Brussel Sprouts, Short Grain and Wild Rice, Quinoa, Leafy Greens (kale, spinach, swiss chard), Bran, Shredded Wheat (unrefined), Sprouted Grains

Golden Rule # 6:

Eat fibrous foods and drink plenty of water for a healthier digestive track. Keeping waste (shit) in your colon is toxic and can lead to cancer.

Man Rule #7

Eat Your Organic Veggies and Fruit, Every day.

Your mommy was right the whole time when she said, *"Eat all your spinach and veggies to grow up big and strong"!*

Most dudes still just like to mow on meat and potatoes. Are you a meat and potato kind of guy?

"Dude, look at me. I'm ripped, I don't eat veggies!" no you're a girly man. There are many bodybuilders out there who look picture perfect. Yet, internally their arteries, organs and blood are not healthy. in Chinese medicinal terms, they are "acidic". So, you're an acidic, ripped girly man.

 Man Tip: find a few veggies you like and buy them frozen. Spend a few extra cents and buy only organic brands. Frozen veggies are great to heat up for a quick meal or snack. Find a dressing you love, natural dressing of course and put mix it in if you don't like the taste of straight up veggies.

Best Veggies To Eat (organic):
Artichoke hearts, Asparagus, Edamame, Broccoli, Brussel Sprouts, Cabbage, Carrots, Cauliflower, Spinach, Kale, Celery, Sauerkraut, Leeks, Peppers, Zucchini, Cucumber, Turnips

Best Fruits to Eat (buy organic):

All Berries, Green Apples, Ripe Bananas, Grapefruit, Mango, Pineapple, Apricots, Watermelon, Cherries, Nectarines, Oranges

Are bananas ok?

Yellower they are, the more sugar they have. Go for slightly greener bananas and you'll get lots of potassium and less sugar. Keep bananas to a minimum. A few slices mashed on a piece of Ezekiel Toast is great with raw nut butter as a snack or even a breakfast to go. They are great to add bulk to a smoothie too.

What is the ORAC Score?

Basically, the Orac score gives you an indication of how a given veggie or fruit fights off free radicals. Free radicals break down all your good cells and create havoc in your body. So, *the more you eat veggies and fruits, the more your body is able to fight free radicals.* Berries have a high Orac score. So, eat berries as much as possible.

Do you believe in the Glycemic Type Diet?

The glycemic index, or gi is a measure of the effects of carbohydrates in food on blood sugar levels. It estimates how much each gram of available carbohydrate (total carbohydrate minus fiber) in a food raises a person's blood glucose level following consumption of the food, relative to consumption of glucose. http://www.glycemic.com/glycemicindex-Loaddefined.htm

Yes, I truly believe that a diet that consist of foods that have a high glycemic index leads to low energy, a big gut, a whole shit load of medical issues and bad results.

That's why if you want six pack abs and lose some weight fast, then you should go eliminate all refined sugars from your diet and even keep complex carbs to a minimum until you see results. Remember, complex carbs are key for an intense workout the next day (heavy weights, sprinting, boxing etc.

Man Rule #8

Eat Like a Hippie

Do you have any of the conditions below:

- ✓ gas
- ✓ acne
- ✓ Pains and arthritis
- ✓ serious fat-shit syndrome
- ✓ no energy
- ✓ erectile dysfunction
- ✓ girl Like qualities

You should completely stay away from the all-American, carb Loaded, fat induced, salt ridden, alcoholic slurping diet.

Yep, you'll have to go green.

You should avoid meats and choose fish and eggs. Focus on veggies, greens, supplements and eat no sugar. Yes, that includes cane sugar, agave, honey, syrup…

Drink lots of water and organic veggie juice.

I could go on with this topic but this book is for those guys who want to eat a healthier all American-fat-boy diet.

Man Rule #9

Sleep is Crucial for Muscle Development and Weight loss

Sleep is very important for your health and muscle development. I really don't want to get into the science of sleep. Simply, rest up.

Food Stuff You Need To Stay Fit

Now, you have the basics above. Let me show you some short-cuts to create food that will fit into your busy lifestyle. This is how I've been able to stay between 7% to 10% body fat at 46 years old.

This is for guys who are on the go and want to keep fit. If, all of the sudden you get the urge to stick a thong up your ass and start posing up on stage, then you're on your own. Just boil chicken, bake some yams, store it in containers and call it a day.

MANLY COOKING TIPS

Cooking healthy food is the key to losing weight, staying young and a great way to get in a girls pants. You can work out all you want, but if you're eating processed, artificial food, then you'll never get the results you expect.

"EAT SHIT. YOU'LL LOOK AND FEEL LIKE SHIT!"
-Doug Bennett

PROTEIN: COOKING TIPS TO SAVE TIME AND MONEY

As you know by now, you need to eat protein to build hard and dense muscles. So, you need it on hand ready to eat. Cook up extra for the week. You can always freeze some of it.

Free-Range chicken/steak: grab a super-sized plastic zip-lock bag and throw steak or chicken in it along with your favorite chemical-free natural dressing (Whole Foods Market has the best selection of rubs and marinades). Try a few and stick with 2-3 you like.

Put it in the fridge for at least an hour, or go crazy and keep it marinating for 24 hours. Remove the meat, throw out the marinade and grill, roast, bake, or stir-fry the meat in a hot pan.

Hard-Boiled eggs: get a giant pot. Boil up enough water to cover all the eggs throw them into the water and place on high heat. Once the water boils, turn it down to simmer twelve minutes from the time of boiling should give you perfect hardboiled eggs. Let them cool down and throw into the fridge.

Eggs for egg sandwiches: whip up 1.5 dozen egg whites and 4 eggs. Pour them into a nice shallow 1 inch pan. Bake for 15 minutes on 350. Cut into squares. Place the eggs in a lettuce wrap or on Ezekiel English muffins/Toast, or better yet without any bread.

Natural Turkey Bacon: Place 16 slices evenly on 2 large baking sheets. Bake each side for 3-8 minutes on 350 degrees.

Beans: pinto, lentils, black, kidney etc....yes they are good for you. Add a few of these to any salad, protein or brown rice. Screw boiling these. Simply, buy the premade organic brand in a can. Rinse them off and you're good to go. I personally only eat lentils.

Ground turkey, chicken or beef: ready to build some muscle: purchase natural, 93% lean ground meat. Whip a few pounds into a large pot with a touch of water and a cover. Break it up as it cooks and fry this stuff up till done.

Ways to eat ground meat once cooked:
- ✓ Combine with brown rice, peas and nuts
- ✓ Mix in 2 tbsp. organic apricot preserves (per pound of chicken or turkey), nuts and dried cranberries.
- ✓ Place on top of Baked Potato with salsa or favorite marinara (no sugar, natural)
- ✓ Cover with Favorite tomato sauce (RAO"S) and Romano
- ✓ Place cold over greens and top with favorite dressing.

Create Your Own Bowl To Take On The Road:

Slap 1-2 cups of ground meat into a big bowl so you can mix any or all of the foods below into it:

- **Starch:** Pre-made brown rice, grilled sweet potato, chopped red potatoes, quinoa
- **Any and all veggies** (kale, broccoli, sweet potato baby spinach, carrots, parsnips ,asparagus...see veggie section above)
- **Nuts and Seeds:** almonds, pumpkin seeds, cashews
- **Fruit:** berries, tomatoes, etc.
- **Natural Dried Fruit:** raisins, dried cranberries, etc.

Stir up, mix it, Beat the shit out of it.....throw into a Tupper Ware container and bring some of your favorite dressing to add into it.

Sweet potato, golden potato, carrot and root veggies mix: always buy these organic! Wash them in a colander. Keep the skin on and chop them up into squares.

Chop them up, boil them until slightly tender. Place them into a pan with extra virgin olive oil and fry them up with sea salt and flavors of your choice (parsley, cayenne pepper, etc.)

Short Grain Brown Rice, Quinoa, Basmati Rice or Wild Rice: cook or buy them frozen at Trader Joes or Whole Foods Market. Once cooked fry in large pot with little olive oil, garlic, salt, chopped onion, chopped carrots, chopped broccoli and add egg white or an egg or two. Those who are lifting too build mass should be eating 2-3 cups of rice and protein after every heavy lift. You can up your intake of 1-2 cups of rice 2-4x day. Note: only if you're lifting heavy and trying to build mass and/or a triathlete.

Barley or Bulger Wheat: no big secret here. Just double the recipe and follow the directions. Quinoa, Barley and Bulger Wheat are all great to add to salads, veggies and soups

Sweet potato, golden potato, carrot and root veggies mix: always buy these organic! Wash them in a colander. Keep the skin on and chop them up into squares.

Chop them up, boil them until slightly tender. Place them into a pan with extra virgin olive oil and fry them up with sea salt and flavors of your choice (parsley, cayenne pepper, etc.)

Short Grain Brown Rice, Quinoa, Basmati Rice or Wild Rice: cook or buy them frozen at Trader Joes or Whole Foods Market. Once cooked fry in large pot with little olive oil, garlic, salt, chopped onion, chopped carrots, chopped broccoli and add egg white or an egg or two. Those who are lifting too build mass should be eating 2-3 cups of rice and protein after every heavy lift. You can up your intake of 1-2 cups of rice 2-4x day. Note: only if you're lifting heavy and trying to build mass and/or a triathlete.

Barley or Bulger Wheat: no big secret here. Just double the recipe and follow the directions. Quinoa, Barley and Bulger Wheat are all great to add to salads, veggies and soups

Fresh Peppers, Spinach, Greens, Tomatoes, Cucumber, Sprouts, Red Onions, Broccoli, Carrots: Wash, cut and chop. Throw into a storage container. Now, you're salad ready. Simply, mix this batch into freshly cut mixed greens and you're good to go.

Condiments, dressing and herbs: condiments, dressing and herbs are key to making simple food taste better.

Herbs: Add fresh herbs while cooking protein or add to starches while cooking. i.e cilantro, parsley, thyme, cinnamon.
Cilantro mixed with ground turkey and pico de gallo.

Dressings: make sure all dressing are preservative free and lower in sugar if possible. Don't worry about a little sugar unless you're getting up on stage to pose the next day, diabetic or weighing in for competition.

NOTE: don't eat any foods with sugar if you're trying to do a complete sugar detox.

I.e. Organic white or red balsamic vinegar, Newman's Own Lite Balsamic or Caesar Dressing, Amy's Teriyaki Marinade.

Condiments: condiments can be helpful to making bland foods tasty. I.e. organic apricot preserves, Earth Balance Butter Spread (no soy), unsweetened organic ketchup. You can have 1-2 tbsps. Of natural barbeque sauce if you're lifting and not worry about it ruining your girly physique. Lift heavier.

THINK YOU HAVE LOWER TESTOSTERONE?

If you think your levels are determined to be on the low side, there are some natural ways to help them.

- Increase your rest and sleep time.
- Eat more complex carbs after lifting heavy or *training in a high endurance activity.
- Lose weight and body fat.
- Add a Medium Chain Triglyceride Oil to your protein shakes, hot cereals, salads, veggies or any other food you prefer. I personally add Udo's 3.6.9 blend to my protein drink and raw coconut oil to my oatmeal or veggies.
- Limit or eliminate alcohol
- -Lift Heavy
- Add intensity to your workouts (sprinting, boxing, etc.)*
- Review any medications your currently on with your doctor.
- Consume a daily probiotic vitamin and mineral
- **Eat healthy Fats

*You can simply increase your T levels by not overtraining.

Many triathletes will improve their T Levels and strength by cutting back or resting an extra day.

** Many of the diets that are on the Internet contain high amounts of saturated fat. However, this increases your calorie intake substantially, which may lead to excess body fat. So, yes eat some fats (20-30%), but screw these diets that call for 50% or even 70% of your diet from healthy fats like olive oil, avocado, coconut oil and raw nuts.

Instead, eat more complex carbs like yams, short grain brown rice and quinoa, which will increase your muscles' glucose levels so you can have a workout that's intense and strong the next day.

WHO DEFINES YOU?

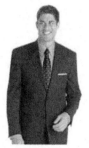

Guy 1 (MONEY GUY):

You care about very little other than being successful and making lots of money. Better yet, you really don't think about what you put into your mouth and sometimes you forget to eat. You eat too few calories or when you do, it's an excessive amount at dinner meetings or late night. Which has led to your skinny frame or your fat dumpy man-tits.

Mission:

Lose belly fat. Build muscle, and improve your fitness. Squeeze in workouts between your family and work. No excuses. Make all of the protein options on a free day or in between manicuring your nails and shaving. Plus, make healthier choices when out in business dinners and luncheons.

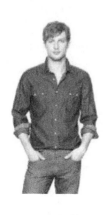

Guy # 2 (LADY KILLER)

You're hoping to get buff so guys think you're tough and the girls want to lick your abs.

Unfortunately, your body doesn't respond to working out like the body of a younger guy.

So, you'll have to work out with intensity and stay strict on a clean diet. Unfortunately, you'll have to eat close to being a thong poser, but without doing steroids. Just like guys # 1 and guys # 3, you'll need to prep for the week and load up with protein. Oh yeah, your training requires a gym. No living room workouts for you.

Mission: build some mass with food and heavy weights, then cut back on the eating and hit the road to make those muscles pop. Stop guzzling the beer and start powering through the workouts I have written for you. You'll need to do some cardio. Nothing is worse than a guy who looks fit but can't jog a mile. Don't be a poser.

Guy #3 (sports guy)

You gave up your workouts and favorite sport to focus on work. You were once a solid player, but you've taken so much time off you're

scared you'll embarrass yourself and get hurt. Now you're ready to get back working out and playing your favorite sport.

Mission:

You should focus on dropping some weight, increasing your stamina and building muscle. We have to get you back into a competitive mind set both at the table as well in the weight room.

THE DIETS

Below are some diet suggestions based upon the guy you have chosen above.

Diet Suggestions

(Guy 1 and 3)

Breakfast Suggestions
Drink Water with Fresh Lemon Juice!

- ✓ Scrambled Egg whites (3-6) dependent on your weight and workout schedule. The more you weight and the harder you train, the more egg whites you should eat. 1-2 cup fresh fruit.
- ✓ Scrambled Egg white omelets with chopped protein (natural turkey bacon, chicken or turkey sausage, grilled chicken or lean steak)
- ✓ Food For Life Ezekiel English Muffin toasted with Raw Almond Butter and 2-3 slices banana smashed onto it. Green Apple
- ✓ Organic Cottage Cheese with added berries and nuts. Optional: add 2-3 slices chopped turkey bacon
- ✓ Grilled steak , egg and fruit
- ✓ Organic Chicken or Turkey Sausage (1-4) with egg whites and tomato
- ✓ 2-4 Scoops Natural Protein Powder blended with beverage (organic unsweetened almond or coconut milk), ½ cup frozen

fruit (berries best) Optional: add tsp raw nut butter, chia seeds, hemp seeds, flax seeds, greens (I personally use the "Super Greens Energy Blend" from Whole Foods Market)

✓ Quinoa Or Oat bowl with raw nuts, seeds (flax, hemp or chia), natural dried fruit, fresh fruit

✓ Plain Greek Yogurt or Organic Low-fat Cottage Cheese with one or all (fresh fruit, dried fruit, raw nuts, protein powder, coconut, "Super Greens Energy Blend from Whole Foods Market", organic oats)

✓ 1-2 Cups Fresh Fruit (mango, pineapple, blueberries) topped with chia seeds, raw nuts and unsweetened vanilla almond milk.

✓ 1-2 cups Ezekiel almond cereal or Barbara's Shredded Wheat with 2% milk or unsweetened almond or coconut milk, ½ cup fresh fruit.

✓ Kale, spinach, tomato, 2 ounces low-fat natural cheese and 1 egg, 3-5 egg white omelet.

✓ Barbara's Shredded Wheat with 3-5 slices banana, organic fruit (buy frozen and defrost i.e. mango) with organic unsweetened almond or coconut milk

✓ Ezekiel Toast or English muffin with one or all of the following: raw almond butter, natural fruit preserves, Earth Balance Butter Spread, Spectrum Oils, and Smashed Banana

✓ Organic Greens with 1-2 eggs over easy on top. Fresh Fruit.

✓ Scrambled ground protein (chicken, beef, turkey, or bison) with egg whites and spinach.

✓ Egg sandwich with Ezekiel English muffin, free-range turkey bacon, egg whites and low-fat cheese.

✓ Organic Green Apple with raw almond butter and low-fat organic cottage cheese.

✓ Green Drink (kale, spinach, Carrot juice etc...) You can make your own or buy one at your local juice bar. 3-4 ounces raw nuts and Greek Yogurt plain.

✓ Protein Drink (2-4 scoops, see above under protein info) with tbsp. raw nut butter or seeds (hemp or flax), ½ cup frozen fruit (all berries, mango, pear), ½ slightly ripe banana, unsweetened almond milk or coconut water. Optional: add 1 or all: Green Powder (Whole Foods Green Energy Blend), ¼ cup organic oats or ½ cup cooked sweet potato, 1 cup kale or spinach.

- ✓ Sweet potato home fries with 2-6 egg whites or 1-3 eggs and natural turkey bacon or lean steak.
- ✓ Organic Oatmeal (quick oats) mixed with a tablespoon oat bran, fresh fruit and tsp. natural cane sugar or agave.
- ✓ **Lundberg** Brown Rice Cake with raw nut butter and natural preserves (no sugar)
- ✓ Egg whites (3-4) scrambled with organic deli turkey or chicken 2-3 slices, tomato and avocado or slice provolone

How about buying breakfast on the road?
Starbuck's right now is the only place that's just ok. Eating out should be your last choice. Starbuck's oatmeal, and egg and cheese on an English muffin is ok once in a while.

You're better off mixing protein powder with coconut water or milk and having raw nuts or a nut bar (Kind Bar) and fresh fruit.

Best Breakfast when eating out: eggs and fruit.

Foods to 100% avoid:
Breads, cereals, baked goods

Condiments:
Organic Ketchup, Hot Sauce, Salsa, Sea Salt, Earth Balance Butter (non-soy), Trader Joes Spicy Peanut Vinaigrette found in the fridge section (great on eggs and ground meat)

Mid-Morning and Mid-Afternoon Snacks Suggestions Drink Water!

✓ Chopped up raw or steamed veggies

✓ 3-6 organic, natural turkey slices from Whole Foods Market, 1 ounce parmesan cheese

✓ Organic Chicken Soup with rice (make your own or find a natural, organic free-range option at Whole Foods Market or Buy The Whole Foods Market, Fresh Homemade Chicken Soup.

✓ Green Apple with raw nut butter

✓ 3-6 slices organic and/or free range deli slices (turkey or chicken breast) and slice natural cheese. Green Apple

✓ Sandwich: 2 slices toasted Ezekiel Muffin filled with 4-8 ounces organic, lean protein: chicken breast, steak, burger (bison, turkey, chicken, beef), organic turkey breast slices and veggies

✓ Fresh Fruit and Plain Greek Yogurt (limit to 1-2 per day)

✓ Lundberg Brown Rice Cake with Almond Butter and Banana Slices or Low-fat Cottage Cheese or Natural Turkey Slices and tomato

✓ 1 hard-boiled egg, 3-5 egg whites with hot sauce or BBQ sauce (make sure its all natural and no preservatives)

✓ Raw Peanut Butter, Natural Preserves on Slice Toasted Ezekiel Sprouted Bread.

✓ Toasted Ezekiel Bread with Avocado, Turkey Bacon Tomato, Sprouts, Lemon Juice and Extra Virgin Olive Oil (limit to 1-2x week).

✓ Protein Drink (2-4 Scoops Protein Powder, Liquid and shake. Fruit only if you didn't have a protein drink with fruit earlier).

✓ 3-8 ounces meat (grilled chicken, steak or turkey) or fish

✓ 1-2 tbsp. raw nut butter (almond or organic peanut butter), green apple

✓ Tuna (1-2 cans) in vegetable broth or water. **My favorite: Starkist** light tuna in sunflower oil in the convenient packet.

Very tasty and you don't need anything in it. Mix with greens or anything. No need for dressing.

✓ 2-4 ounces Raw nuts and natural dried fruit

✓ Nut bar if you're on the road (Kind Bar is ok once in a while if no alternative. Skip all other bars unless organic raw food bar)

✓ 2 Brown rice cakes (Lundberg Brand), piece of fruit or cup organic berries

✓ 1-2 cups brown or wild rice with 1 once nuts, seed and/or dried fruit

✓ Organic (must be all natural!!) turkey, beef or bison jerky. Green apple

✓ Sweet Potato or Baked Potato with salsa or tsp Earth Balance Butter or Low-Fat Cottage Cheese.

✓ Veggie stir fry with chicken

✓ Sushi (no artificial flavors or ingredients) I purchase from Whole foods.

✓ Plain Greek Yogurt (add fresh fruit, raw nuts and dried fruit. My favorite: dried cranberries, fresh blueberries, pumpkin seeds, almonds, walnuts)

✓ Piece of Fruit (orange, green apple)

✓ Organic Chicken Soup or Broth Soup with added Protein

✓ Green Drink (local juice bar)

Lunch (Midday) Suggestions
Drink water!

✓ 1-2 cups wild or brown rice (1/2 cup white rice), 4-8 ounces of protein, mixed greens with dressing

✓ Organic soup (protein included or a lentil/bean soup), mixed greens with natural dressing

✓ Bowls: mix all together/options: 1-2 cups steamed or raw veggies (always kale and spinach If possible), 1 cup starch (rice, sweet potato, regular potato, root veggies, udon or brown rice noodles), dairy (½ cup low-fat organic cottage cheese, 1 ounce low-fat natural cheese), 2 ounces seeds and/or nuts. See my favorite in recipes.

- ✓ 4-8 ounces sushi (raw tuna or fish, no mayo based and always all natural), sea weed salad, mixed greens and/or 1 cup fruit
- ✓ Green Drink (local juice bar), 2-4 ounces raw nuts, 1 cup Plain Greek Yogurt, piece of organic fruit.
- ✓ 3-6 ounces natural turkey or chicken deli slices on Engine 21 hamburger roll with slice natural cheese and toppings (lettuce, tomato, cukes). My favorite dressing: tbsp. organic apricot preserves with ½ tsp organic mustard or organic, natural spicy bbq sauce.
- ✓ 1 cup pasta (brown rice, **Tinkyada Brand** or wheat is best) mixed with 1-3 cups lean, free-range and/or organic meat (buffalo, beef, chicken, turkey)
- ✓ Protein Drink mixed with tbsp. nut butter, 1-2 hard-boiled eggs.
- ✓ Mexican Bowl: brown rice, greens, beef or chicken, salsa, cilantro, tsp. avocado. No beans
- ✓ Plain Tuna with greens, Paul Newman's Light Italian or Oil and Vinegar dressing, greens, tomato, sliced peppers and cucumbers placed between Ezekiel Toast. Piece of Fruit.
- ✓ Lettuce Wrap, Trader Joes Spicy Peanut Vinaigrette mixed with 4-8 ounces grilled chicken, steak, fish or ground protein. Piece of fruit.
- ✓ Protein Drink (2-4 scoops, see above under protein info) with tbsp. raw nut butter or seeds (hemp or flax), ½ cup frozen fruit (all berries, mango, pear), ½ slightly ripe banana, unsweetened almond milk or coconut water. Optional: add 1 or all: Green Powder (Whole Foods Green Energy Blend), ¼ cup organic oats or ½ cup cooked sweet potato, 1 cup kale or spinach.
- ✓ 1-2 cups chicken soup and small piece sourdough bread. 1 Cup or Piece Fruit.
- ✓ 4-8 Ounces Grilled chicken, 1-2 cups green beans, broccoli, peas and brown rice.

- ✓ 1 egg, 3-6 egg white scramble or omelet with spinach, shitake mushrooms sweet potato and broccoli all mixed in. (optional: add low-fat cheese on top), Greek Yogurt.
- ✓ Stir fry: 4-8 ounces protein with 1-2 cups veggies. Mixed greens with vinegar and oil.
- ✓ 4-8 ounces protein (steak, turkey, chicken, and tuna) wrapped in Boston Bibb Lettuce with veggies of choice. 1-2 Cups Starch (brown rice, wild rice, etc.)
- ✓ 1-2 scoops Whole Foods Green Energy Blend mixed with unsweetened almond milk, 3-4 ounces raw nuts and piece of fruit.
- ✓ Organic chicken or veggie soup (you can buy soups at your local market in the natural food section or whole foods), greens and piece of fruit.
- ✓ 4-8 ounces Protein on salad greens mixed with nuts and cottage cheese. Protein drink with 1-2 scoops protein powder.

Still hungry?
- ✓ If you're trying to lose weight, drink Water or tea with lemon and suck it up. Go cry.
- ✓ If you're a skinny weed and trying to gain weight, than double your calorie intake by increasing your protein by 2-3 ounces, fat by 1-2 ounces and carbs 1-2 cups but make sure you train hard or all those extra calories will go to stored fat or you'll just shit them out.

Dinner Suggestions
Drink Water!

NOTE: I suggest eating a little more protein if and only if you're lifting heavy to help your muscles at night repair while you sleep. If you're trying to lose weight, keep your protein portions between 4-6 ounces dependent on your weight and take a branched chain amino acid supplement.

- ✓ 5-12 ounces fish, baked potato, mixed greens and veggies with extra virgin olive oil and lemon.
- ✓ 2-3 cups sautéed veggies with 5-10 ounces cooked protein (ground buffalo, sliced steak, chopped chicken). Mix all in with 1 cup quinoa, wild rice or brown rice pasta. Put parmesan or your favorite dressing on top i.e. **Trader Joes Spicy Peanut Vinaigrette**, Coconut oil and pepper, Hot Sauce, Tomato Sauce (unsweetened), Herbs (parsley, cilantro).
- ✓ Broiled free-range chicken on the bone, sautéed spinach, 1-2 cups brown rice or sweet potato. Mixed greens with Paul Newman's Light Dressing or see my dressings.
- ✓ 1 Cup Brown Rice pasta or udon noodles with sautéed veggies, 5-10 ounces steamed chicken, Bragg's Liquid Aminos (1-2tsps.). Mixed Greens
- ✓ 5-10 ounces Lean Steak, steamed spinach or favorite veggies, baked potato
- ✓ 1-2 cups of Cauliflower rice (found at Whole Foods or Trader Joes), Mixed with cooked 5- 10 ounces ground turkey and broccoli placed over greens and topped with all natural low-fat regular or dairy free ranch or poppy seed dressing.
- ✓ 1x week: 2-4 Slices Thin Crust Pizza (make sure you buy from a restaurant that uses only fresh foods) topped with chicken and veggies. Mixed Greens with nuts.
- ✓ Tacos: 6-14 ounces lean ground protein (buffalo, chicken, beef, and turkey) or fish placed in hard organic, stone taco shells (find in natural food section, Whole Foods or Trader Joes), Slices avocado, lettuce, low-fat cheese and fresh Pico De Gallo or favorite hot sauce. Mixed greens.
- ✓ 8-12 ounces Shredded Chicken Breast with chopped broccoli (steamed), mixed with extra virgin olive oil, lemon juice, pine nuts, parsley and parmesan cheese.
- ✓ 1-2: 8 ounce bean and oat, Buffalo or Lean Beef Burger with sautéed shitake mushrooms, onions and turkey bacon placed between toasted Ezekiel English Muffin. Top with organic

ketchup or favorite hot sauce. Sweet potato fries (broil each side till crisp) or baked potato. Mixed greens.

✓ 1-2 Cups Brown Rice or Wheat pasta mixed with 1-2 cups cooked ground protein or top with a over easy cooked egg, sautéed garlic, fresh parsley, walnuts, extra virgin olive or coconut oil and dash organic balsamic vinegar with ¼ cup low-fat mozzarella.

✓ 1-2 cups of Ceviche, mixed greens and 1-2 cups wild rice.

✓ 3-8 protein meatballs placed on top of rice or pasta with or without favorite natural tomato sauce (unsweetened).

✓ 1-3 cups of soup (home-made chicken and rice, lemon and chicken, veggie soup, turkey chicken or lean beef chili) 1-2 slices Ezekiel Toast with Earth Balance Butter. Mixed Greens.

✓ Green Drink with 2-4 scoops hemp protein. 1-3 cup sautéed veggies (root veggies, broccoli, kale, peas) placed into 1- 2 cups free range chicken broth or organic veggie broth and mixed greens.

Supplements to Take at Night:

Always consult Your Medical Professional Before Taking Supplement.

✓ Pro-biotic Daily Multiple Vitamin
✓ 1800 mg Branched Chain Aminos
✓ 1000 mg Vitamin C

GUY 2

Breakfast Suggestions

*Sorry buddy, you'll have to eat more like your thong wearing body builder buddy

Breakfast
Drink Water!

- ✓ Scrambled Egg whites (4-8) dependent on your weight and workout schedule. The more you weight and the harder you train, the more egg whites you should eat. 1-2 cups oatmeal
- ✓ Scrambled Egg white omelets (3-4) with chopped protein (natural turkey bacon, chicken or turkey sausage, grilled chicken or lean steak). 1-2 cups organic cottage cheese
- ✓ 4-8 ounces chicken or steak with 1-2 eggs or 2-4 egg whites. 1-2 cups Greek Yogurt
- ✓ 3-5 slices Natural Turkey bacon. 1-2 cups Sweet Potato Home Fries. 1 cup Cottage Cheese or 2 hard-boiled eggs
- ✓ 1-2 cups basmati brown rice mixed with 4-5 egg whites, 1-2 turkey bacon and top with parmesan cheese and/or tbsp. organic apricot preserves mixed in well.
- ✓ 1-2 cups Ezekiel almond cereal or Barbara's Shredded Wheat with 2% milk, ½ cup fresh fruit. 1- 2 cups low-fat organic cottage cheese.
- ✓ Protein drink: 2-4 scoops favorite protein with ½ cup frozen organic fruit and 2% milk or unsweetened almond milk. 1-2 cups Barbara's Shredded Wheat.

✓ Broiled or Grilled Chicken 4-6 ounces, 2-3 Egg Whites all mixed with fresh Pico De Gallo and low-fat cheese (2-3 ounces). Slice Ezekiel Toast

✓ 1-2 fried eggs, 2 slices Ezekiel toast with Earth Balance Butter Spread, Sweet Potato home fries, Turkey bacon

✓ 1-2 cups cooked organic oats, tsp natural cane sugar or coconut sugar, fresh fruit. Protein drink

✓ 1-2 cups organic oats with fresh fruit (ORGANIC blueberries, strawberries). Handful raw nuts. 1 Cup Organic Low-fat Cottage Cheese

✓ 3-6 egg hard-boiled egg whites, 1-2 tbsp. raw nut butter on brown rice cake with apple butter on top.

✓ 2-4 Egg Whites between Toasted Ezekiel English Muffin with 3-5 slices Natural Turkey Bacon, tomato. 1 cup berries or green apple.

✓ 3-5 Egg whites, 1 fried egg, 5-8 ounces natural sirloin steak tips

✓ Toasted Ezekiel Egg White (3-6 egg whites, 1 egg) Sandwich with organic salsa on top.

NOTE: Turkey bacon may have 200 mg of salt per slice, so if you're on a low-salt diet than I would axe the turkey bacon slices. Just sayin…

Mid-Morning and Mid-Afternoon Snacks
Drink Water!

✓ Chopped up raw or steamed veggies

✓ Egg White (3-6 egg whites, 1 egg) with broccoli or spinach (buy Frozen organic chopped spinach or broccoli, microwave and mix with egg whites) add hot sauce (My favorite is Trader Joe's Green Dragon).

✓ Organic Chicken Soup with rice (find a natural, organic free-range option at Whole Foods Market or Buy **The Whole Foods Market**, Fresh Homemade Chicken Soup.

- ✓ Green Apple with raw nut butter. 5-8 slices Natural Turkey Bacon or Natural, Organic Turkey Breast from Whole Foods Market
- ✓ 1-2 Cups ground, lean meat (my favorite: natural bison) with ½ - 1 cup brown rice pasta shells or 1-2 cups broccoli or spinach (buy Frozen organic chopped spinach or broccoli, microwave and mix with egg whites) and Romano or Parmesan cheese.(Optional: RAO's Marinara)
- ✓ Tuna (1-2 cans) in vegetable broth or water. **My favorite: Starkist** light tuna in sunflower oil in the convenient packet. Very tasty and you don't need anything in it. Mix with greens or anything. No need for dressing.
- ✓ Fresh Fruit and Low-Fat Organic Cottage Cheese (must be organic)
- ✓ Salad Greens with cucumbers, sprouts, ½ cup low-fat cottage cheese, dried fruit, nuts, seeds carrots, 3-8 ounces protein or beans and your favorite dressing (lemon juice, tsp oil, sea salt and pepper) or low-fat natural dressing.
- ✓ Protein Drink (2-4 Scoops Protein Powder, Liquid and shake. Fruit only if you didn't have a protein drink with fruit earlier).
- ✓ 3-8 ounces meat (grilled chicken, steak or turkey) or fish. Plain Greek Yogurt or Low-fat Cottage Cheese. Skip both if you had either for breakfast. Replace with handful raw nuts.
- ✓ 1-2 cups of lentils and 1 cup of rice, chopped herbs and onion, tsp. Earth Balance Butter
- ✓ *1-2 Can(s) tuna in vegetable broth or water, green apple
- ✓ 1-2 cups steamed or raw spinach, kale mixed with organic lentils (buy frozen or in can and rinse well). Optional: Place cheese or marinara or favorite natural dressing on top.
- ✓ 1 cup Raw nuts and natural dried fruit, 1 cup organic Low-Fat cottage cheese
- ✓ Brown rice cake (Lundberg Brand) with 2 tbsp raw nut butter
- ✓ 1-2 cups brown or wild rice with 2 ounces nuts, seed and ½ -1 cup ground meat

✓ Organic (must be all natural!!) turkey, beef or bison jerky. Green apple

✓ Sweet Potato or Baked Potato with ½-1 cup ground meat, egg whites or Low-Fat Cottage Cheese. Top with salsa or balsamic vinegar. If chicken, turkey or egg whites try with 1 tbsp. organic apricot preserves mixed into all.

✓ 1-3 cups Veggie stir fry with chicken or meat

✓ Raw Fish Sushi (no artificial flavors or ingredients) with or without brown rice.

✓ 1 cup Plain Greek Yogurt or Organic Low-fat Cottage Cheese (add fresh fruit, raw nuts and dried fruit. My favorite: dried cranberries, fresh blueberries, pumpkin seeds, almonds, walnuts)

✓ Piece of Fruit (orange, green apple), 4-8 ounces grilled chicken

✓ Protein Drink (2 scoops natural whey or hemp protein), ½ cup frozen fruit and unsweetened almond milk

✓ *limit you're canned tuna intake to 2-4 servings per week due to high mercury intake. Science has proven that these types of fishes may contain excess mercury.

Lunch Suggestion
DRINK WATER!

Alright bucket head, this is when shit gets a little bland. Yet, you want to impress the guys with bulging biceps and want to have abs for the ladies right? Fortunately, for you, your diet won't be as plain as your thong wearing buddy.

✓ 6 – 12 ounces ground meat with 1 cup brown or even white rice mixed well and topped with tsp Organic Coconut oil or tsp. Earth Balance Butter. Mixed Greens with chopped fruit

✓ 6- 12 ounces broiled chicken on the bone, ½ - 1 cup home fries or baked potato (sweet or red bliss), ½ cup organic low-fat cottage cheese

✓ 2-3 Broiled chicken thighs, 1-2 cups brown rice mixed with peas and/or broccoli, 1-2 cups steamed spinach

✓ Ground chicken or turkey, brown rice, steamed broccoli and nuts with favorite sauce : i.e. organic apricot preserves, natural ranch dressing, hot sauce.

✓ 6-12 ounces protein (fish, chicken, beef, turkey) on top of mixed greens with nuts, seeds, low-fat cottage cheese, berries and yams or 1 cup rice

✓ Protein Drink 2-4 scoops protein (hemp or whey), ½ cup frozen fruit, 1 tbsp. raw nut butter and ¼ cup oats. 1 cup low-fat milk is ok.

✓ 1-2 cups lean protein chili and 1 cup rice, mixed greens

✓ 6-16 ounces burger wrapped in lettuce or on top of salad greens. Baked potato. Veggies.

✓ Kale salad with extra virgin olive oil, walnuts or almonds, berries, tomatoes and topped with 8-16 ounces of fish (halibut, cod, salmon or tuna)

✓ Raw Tuna Roll (8-12 ounces), Mixed Greens with Veggies

✓ Chicken Soup: place cooked pulled chicken off the bone (2-3 cups) and place in Organic Chicken Broth with Spinach, Chopped Carrots, ½ cup wild rice, ½ cup yams, 1 cup celery. Boil till all tender. Eat with 1-2 slices toasted Ezekiel toast with Earth Balance butter.

✓ 2 **Starkist** Light Tuna Packets (in sunflower oil) or favorite tuna, mix with spinach or kale, brown rice, tomatoes and cucumbers. Top with Apple Cider Vinegar.

✓ Zucchini Pasta with 6-12 ounces shrimp or chicken mixed with parsley, lemon, parmesan cheese and steamed spinach

✓ 8-12 ounces grilled lean steak with sautéed shitake mushrooms over wild rice 1-2 cups. Mixed Greens and sliced green apple.

✓ 6-12 ounces Chicken and 1-2 cups Broccoli stir-fry mixed with ½ cup brown rice shells or brown basmati rice and low-fat mozzarella or Romano cheese.

✓ **Chipotle:** double meat with brown rice, lettuce, corn, salsa and hot sauce

✓ 1 cup Barley mixed with 12 ounces Ground chicken, buffalo or turkey, dried cranberries, ½ cup raw walnuts and 1-2 cups kale. Top with low-fat organic ranch or Greek Dressing.

✓ **Thai Food:** Small portion Cashew Chicken at your local Thai Food Restaurant (make sure no MSG). 1-3 servings of grilled chicken on the stick

✓ 8-12 ounces protein, 1-2 cups basmati brown rice or potato (sweet or red), 1 cup organic low-fat cottage cheese, 1-2 cups stir fry or steamed veggies

✓ 3 : 4 ounce grilled steak portions with grilled onions and mushrooms in a lettuce wrap. Dip into your favorite marinade or dressing found in natural food section Whole Foods Market. 1 cup rice (white, wild or brown).

Dinner Suggestions
Drink Water!

NOTE: Eat more protein since you're lifting heavy to help your muscles at night repair while you sleep. If you're trying to lose weight, keep your protein portions between 4-6 ounces dependent on your weight and take a branched chain amino acid supplement.

✓ 8-14 ounces fish, 1 baked potato, 1-2 cups mixed greens and veggies with extra virgin olive oil and lemon.

✓ 2-3 cups sautéed veggies with 8-14 ounces cooked protein (ground buffalo, sliced steak, chopped chicken). Mix all in with 1 cup quinoa, wild rice or brown rice pasta. Put parmesan or your favorite dressing on top i.e. **Trader Joes Spicy Peanut Vinaigrette**, Coconut oil and pepper, Hot Sauce, Tomato Sauce (unsweetened), Herbs (parsley, cilantro).

✓ Broiled free-range chicken on the bone (12-16 ounces), sautéed spinach, 1-2 cups brown rice or sweet potato. Mixed greens with Paul Newman's Light Dressing or see my dressings.

✓ 1-2 Cup (s) Brown Rice pasta or udon noodles with sautéed veggies, 8-14 ounces steamed chicken, Bragg's Liquid Aminos (1-2tsps.). Mixed Greens

✓ 8-14 ounces Lean Steak or chicken, 2 cups steamed spinach or favorite veggies,1 baked potato

✓ 1-2 cups of Cauliflower rice (found at Whole Foods or Trader Joes), Mixed with cooked 8- 12 ounces ground turkey and broccoli placed over greens and topped with all natural low-fat regular or dairy free ranch or poppy seed dressing.

✓ 1x week: 2-4 Slices Thin Crust Pizza (make sure you buy from a restaurant that uses only fresh foods) topped with extra chicken and veggies. Mixed Greens with nuts.

✓ Tacos: 8-14 ounces lean ground protein (buffalo, chicken, beef, and turkey) or fish placed in hard organic, stone taco shells (find in natural food section, Whole Foods or Trader Joes), Slices avocado, lettuce, low-fat cheese and fresh Pico De Gallo or favorite hot sauce. Mixed greens.

✓ 8-14 ounces lean protein, 1 cup brown basmati or cauliflower rice, 1-2 cups steamed or stir fry veggies.

✓ 8-14 ounces Shredded Chicken Breast with Shaved Brussel sprouts, mixed with extra virgin olive oil, lemon juice, pine nuts, parsley and parmesan cheese.

✓ 1-2: 8 ounce bean and oat, Buffalo or Lean Beef Burger with sautéed shitake mushrooms, onions and turkey bacon placed between toasted Ezekiel English Muffin. Top with organic ketchup or favorite hot sauce. Sweet potato fries (broil each side till crisp) or baked potato. Mixed greens.

✓ 1-2 Cups Brown Rice or Wheat pasta mixed with 1-2 cups cooked ground protein or top with an over easy cooked egg, sautéed garlic, fresh parsley, walnuts, extra virgin olive or coconut oil and dash organic balsamic vinegar with ¼ cup low-fat mozzarella.

✓ 2-3 cups of Ceviche (see recipe) or raw fish, mixed greens and 1-2 cups wild rice.

- ✓ 5-8 protein meatballs (no flour or pork) placed on top of rice or pasta with or without favorite natural tomato sauce (unsweetened).
- ✓ 2-3 cups of soup (home-made chicken and rice, lemon and chicken, veggie soup, turkey chicken or lean beef chili) 1-2 slices Ezekiel Toast with Earth Balance Butter. Mixed Greens.
- ✓ Protein with 2-4 scoops hemp protein. 2-3 cup sautéed veggies (root veggies, broccoli, kale, peas) placed into 1- 2 cups free range chicken broth or organic veggie broth and mixed greens.

Supplements to Take at Night:

Always consult Your Medical Professional before taking any Supplement.
- ✓ Pro-biotic Daily Multiple Vitamin
- ✓ 3000 mg Branched Chain Aminos
- ✓ 1000 mg Vitamin C

Don't Like My Food Suggestions?

Go fuck yourself. Ha, kidding. I'm sure you're a great guy.

Below, I created 2 simple guides for you to either lose weight or pack on pounds and muscle. Just fill them in with the foods you like. If you need more food than simply add more veggies and/or lean protein.

CAUTION: If you're not working out with weights and/or performing cardio. No diet will help you look good for the

LONG-TERM or get you stronger.

You need resistance workouts to change your muscle definition whether that's training with barbells, picking up rocks, chopping wood, hitting a heavy bag and so on.

WEIGHT LOSS PLAN GUIDE

This is the diet when you're ready to pull your skirt up and just sick of feeling like a fat toad.

Breakfast
- 3-8 ounces protein and 1-2 cups or 1 whole fruit (**Example:** 4-8 egg whites, 2 cups organic blueberries)
- Water

Snack 1
- **Protein Drink:** 2-4 scoops protein mixed with 1 cup frozen fruit, water or nondairy beverage or 3-6 ounces lean protein
- 4-6 ounces raw nuts
- **Example:** 4 scoops whey protein mixed coconut water, 4-6 ounces raw almonds

Lunch
- 2-5 cups salad greens
- 1 cup good starch or organic fruit
- 1 cup veggies
- 6-14 ounces protein

Example:
Power bowl: 1 cup brown rice (instant short grain Trader Joes) mixed with 1 cup steamed broccoli and kale, 12 ounces ground turkey or chicken with parmesan cheese and Trader Joes Green Dragon Hot Sauce on top of greens.

Snack 2
- Water, 8-12 ounces protein
- 1 cup good carbs or Low-fat Cottage Cheese
- 2-4 ounces raw nuts

Example:
8 ounces grilled chicken mixed with 1 cup cauliflower rice, 4 ounces raw almonds and chopped tomatoes and cucumbers. Drizzle tsp coconut oil and vinegar on top

Dinner
- 8-14 ounces protein
- 2 cups veggies
- 2-3 cups salad greens

Example: broiled cod, 2 cups kale and salad with 1-2 tbsp. extra virgin olive oil and white balsamic vinegar

Snack 3:

Optional: 6-8 ounces lean protein

Recommended (nightly):
- 1000 mg Vitamin C
- 1500 mg Branched Chain Amino Acid

MUSCLE- UP DIET

This diet is for those who just want to keep it simple, stupid but build the muscle you desire. You must be training 70-90% of your max at least 4 days per week and enjoy eating frequently. Yes, this is more of a body building diet.

MEAL 1
- 6-8 Egg whites
- 1-2 cups starch (brown jasmine rice or 2 slices Ezekiel toast with Earth Balance or Organic butter.
- Branched chain amino acids 5 grams

MEAL 2
- 6-8 ounces chicken/fish/turkey
- 1-3 cups or 20-40 grams complex carbs (i.e. sweet potato, **Lundberg** brown rice cake, jasmine brown rice)
- 1 cup blueberries or green apple

MEAL 3
- 6-10 ounces chicken/fish/bison
- 1-2 cups Veggies
- 1 cup potato (red bliss or sweet) or rice
  Example: Power Bowl with 8 ounces ground bison, 1 cup jasmine rice, sautéed veggies all mixed up with 1 tsp olive oil and dashes of Trader Joe's Green Dragon hot sauce.
- Branched chain amino acids 5 grams

MEAL 4
- 1 cup Organic Low-Fat Cottage Cheese or Greek Yogurt (plain)
- 2-4 ounces raw nuts

Or

Protein Drink:
- 2-4 scoops Plant Protein, 1 Cup Frozen Berries, Coconut Water or Unsweetened Almond Milk.

MEAL 5
- 6-12 Ounces chicken/fish/turkey/lean beef
- 1-2 cups veggies

- 1-2 cups salad greens with 1 tbsp. good oil (organic), lemon juice.
- Branched Chain Amino Acids 5 grams

Example:
12 ounces Grilled Halibut, 1 cup Grilled Peppers and Broccoli, 2 handfuls of Organic Arugula with 1tbsp. extra virgin olive oil and sea salt.

MEAL 6
Hemp Protein Drink or 7-10 Ounces Protein, ½ cup Good Carbs

Weight Loss Questions Answered

Which diet is best for me?
I'm not you. You figure it out. Take your skirt off and take action. The best diet is one that fits into your lifestyle without starting and stopping some crazy diet plan every other week. Just eat clean and if you fuck up 1 day. No big deal. Make your healthy diet a way of life. The more you eliminate unrefined sugar from your diet, the better.

I'm eating healthy but not losing weight?
Simply cut back on your calories and run your ass off. You became a fat slob because you use food as comfort or you blame it on a breakup, your family or some other poor excuse. It's simple,

"Eat Less and Train Harder! "

To speed things up. Cut Calories by eliminating sugars and fats from your diet. Yes, that includes keeping even fruits to a minimum per day (I suggest sticking with 1-2 cups berries for your fruit source.)

However, you can't stay on this diet forever. Plus, you must train hard.

NOTE: if you have done everything above and are still not seeing results after 4-5 weeks of **consistent** dieting and training. Consult with your doctor for hormone imbalance and therapy.

Should I read all labels?
Yes, even when it's sushi. Many of the prepacked raw fish foods have artificial ingredients. Look out for sugars and preservatives.

What if I have a bad eating day?
Just get back on the gravy train. Get your rubber suit on and start sweating, kidding kind of. Eat a no carb diet for the day and drink water until you start to swish with every step. Next day, get back on your healthy eating plan. Oh yeah, lift heavy.

Is Organic really necessary
Yes and no. Keep it simple. Eat organic fruit and veggies, if you have the choice. Free range and organic meats are also better for you. Buy organic frozen veggies (broccoli, peas, cauliflower, etc.) as they are cheaper and most likely better for you.

Do I have to exercise?
Yes. If you don't attempt to start making all of this part of a lifestyle, then forget everything you've read or learned. Don't

Exercise. Don't eat healthy. Just stick to drinking beer, eating both pork rinds and alfalfa sprouts.

What about pasta and starches?
If you're on a mission to lose a big belly. Cut the pasta for a while or limit quantity (1 cup) @ 1-2 x week until you build muscle. Try variations of pasta: soba noodles, brown rice pasta, gluten-free pasta, egg noodles and spelt pasta. Best advice: lift heavy weights to burn those extra carbs and get a great pump after a heavy carb day.

How much of losing Weight is nutrition?

Exercising, eating healthy and adequate sleep are all important components to losing weight. Nutrition is the major factor to making your muscle grow and pop out.

How much sugar can I eat per day?

Once you begin to decrease your daily sugar intake, you should feel a big difference in your energy, mood and belt loop. Your genetics plays a key role in the way your body deals with sugar. Try to eat sugars that are naturally in fruit and occasionally place natural sweetener in your food. Your body will adjust to a lower sugar diet. Excessive sugar can cause havoc in your body. Actually a diet that's high in sugar can cause great stress to your liver and mimic the same effects of excess alcohol which leads to liver damage.

Cereals?

Cereals are 99% shit. The only cereal I recommend is Ezekiel Almond. Another brand of cereal that is ok if you just need a breakfast cereal is "Natures Path". Again, be careful of flour. Think about what flour looks like before it's baked. Sludge.

RECIPES YOU MAY LIKE

Egg Sandwich

Toasted Ezekiel English muffins or Toast top with any of the following:
- Natural Cheddar cheese (2-3 ounces), 3-5 slices organic turkey bacon and an egg or 2-3 egg whites
- 3-5 slices organic turkey bacon, 2-3 egg whites, slice avocado and lettuce
- Sliced organic avocado, egg and a tomato slice
- 3-5 ounces sirloin and 2-3 egg whites

Organic Oatmeal or Quinoa:

1-2 cups oatmeal or quinoa (select organic quick oats or organic quinoa. Don't eat packaged oatmeal or quick oats found in fast food shops, Dunkin Donuts, Convenient Stores (full of salt and sugar).

Optional Add Ins:
- chopped dates or organic dried fruit (1 ounce)
- ½ cup favorite fruit (berries, sliced banana)
- tsp. of natural maple syrup if you need it
- ounces chopped nut or raw almond butter

Top with organic 2% milk or unsweetened non-dairy beverage (Unsweetened organic: almond, rice, hemp, organic or coconut)

Breakfast
Greek Yogurt or Cottage Cheese

8-12 ounces of an all-natural plain Greek Yogurt or
Organic low fat cottage cheese. Add one or all of the following:

- 2 scoops favorite protein powder
- Tbsp. organic natural preserves (apricot, raspberry)
- ½ cup fresh berries
- 1 small organic banana mashed or sliced up
- 1 ounce raw nuts
- 1 ounce dried fruit

*Cottage cheese must be organic. Regular cottage cheese is loaded with preservatives!

*You can buy premixed raw or all natural dried fruit and nuts. Best mix is dried cranberries, almonds, cashews, pumpkin seeds and walnuts.

Blender Breakfast Smoothie

Ingredients:

- 2-4 scoops natural protein powder (plant based or organic whey)
- 1 cup unsweetened almond or coconut milk or organic 2% milk.
- 1 tbsp. raw nut (almond) butter or hemp, flax and chia seeds
- ½ cup organic frozen fruit

Frozen Fruit Combination Ideas:

- pear, banana, tsp. cinnamon, ½ tsp nutmeg, 2-4 raw dates
- Mango, banana
- Berry mix, banana
- Raspberry, cherry, banana
- Apple, cinnamon, nutmeg, 2-4 dates

Directions:
Blend all ingredients. Blend in protein mix last once all blended on slow speed.

Post-Workout Smoothie

Ingredients:
- 2-4 scoops protein mix
- Coconut water
- ½ cup frozen fruit or ice
- 1 tbsp. MCT (medium chain triglyceride) oil or raw nut butter

Directions:
Blend all ingredients. Blend in protein mix last once all blended on slow speed.

Mediterranean Chicken

Ingredients
- 4 free range chicken quarters (breast or thigh), bone in
- 2 tablespoons of chopped fresh thyme
- 2 cloves of chopped garlic
- 3 tablespoons of extra virgin olive oil
- lemon juice from 3 lemons
- sea salt to taste

Directions:
1. Combine all of the ingredients in a small bowl and mix well.
2. Place into large Zip Lock plastic bag along with chicken quarters. Shake well and marinate in refrigerator for 2 to 4 hours (overnight is always best).
3. Pan fry all ingredients, making sure start with bone facing down for 15 minutes, flip and cook until bone can be easily pulled off the bone approximately 10 minutes.

4. Place cover on top for last 5 minutes to make sure cooked.

Chicken and Potato Italian Style

Must have good red sauce, no sugar (RAOS)

Ingredients:
- 1 lb. Natural Ground Chicken or Turkey, lean
- 1 Jar of Spicy or Regular Marinara (My Favorite Is RAO"S)
- ½ cup shitake 1/2 or sliced mushrooms
- 1 cup Chopped Frozen Organic Spinach
- medium golden yellow organic potatoes

Directions:
1. Sauté ground chicken and break up into small pieces as it cooks. Best way to cook: place in skillet, ¼ cup water and cover on medium heat. As it cooks, break it up and stir. Keep adding water as needed. Once done, drain all water and put to side.
2. Sauté mushrooms and peas until slightly tender. Add back the chicken and mix all. Add the softened potatoes and chop the potatoes until very small and mix all together well on low heat.
3. Add sauce, mix and add ½ cup freshly grated Romano Cheese.

Serve with greens (salad)

RECIPE HACK:
5 INGREDIENT SWEET AND SPICY CHICKEN LETTUCE WRAPS
Sometimes you just don't have the time to make a long ingredient recipe meal. Yes, you could saute' fresh apricots, add soy sauce, hoisin sauce, etc..

Yet, with just the right healthy premade products. You can make a great meal without all the food prep.

Try this easy one that taste yummy in a pinch.

Ingredients:
- 1 lb. organic ground chicken
- 1-2 cups steamed organic broccoli
- 2-3 tbsp. ORGANIC Apricot Preserves (low sugar if possible)
- 1/4 - 1/2 cup raw (optional) nut mix: almonds, cashews, dried cranberries, peanuts
- Trader Joes Green Dragon Hot Sauce (try this one!)
- Boston Lettuce Leafs

Prep:
1. Sauté and dice up ground chicken till thoroughly done. Blend in broccoli and nut mix.
2. Add preserves and stir till all ingredients covered. Drizzle hot sauce to taste and mix all together.

Great even as is with just salad greens and/or wild rice.

Easy Bolognese Paleo Style

Ingredients:
- 1 jar of favorite natural red sauce (RAO'S)
- 16 Ounces Organic Meat (choose: bison, chicken, beef, turkey)
- 1-2 cups cooked cauliflower rice

Procedure:
1. Sauté meal till done.
2. Add Sauce and stir.
3. Mix in cauliflower rice.

Steak & Red Wine reduction

Ingredients:
- 2 cloves sliced garlic
- 2 tbsps. Extra virgin olive oil
- Sea salt and pepper
- 2 cups frozen organic chopped spinach
- 2 – 6 ounce sirloin filets
- ½ cup organic cooking red wine
- 1 small white onion
- 2 tbsps. Thyme
- 1 tsp onion powder

Directions:
1. Sauté garlic, onion and olive oil.
2. Place the steak in pan on high heat and top with onions and garlic. Sear for 5-10 minutes
3. Flip the steak and cook for 2-5 minutes dependent on liking.
4. Place steak aside and in same pan.
5. Pour the red wine into the pan and reduce until slightly thick and add thyme, onion pepper, sea salt and pepper.
6. Steam Spinach in separate pan.
7. Pour the reduction over the steak, sautéed spinach and done!

Serve with wild or organic potato (red or sweet) and salad.

Chicken N' Pasta Wine Style

Ingredients:
- ½ cup organic white wine
- 1 tbsp. sea salt
- 4 cups free range chicken broth
- 1 handful parsley
- 4 tbsps. lemon juice
- 1 tbsp. olive oil

- 1 clove sliced thin garlic
- 16 ounces chopped chicken breast
- 1 cup chopped cherry tomatoes
- 1 cup organic steamed broccoli

Directions:

1. **Sauce:** Simmer first 5 ingredients for 15 minutes.
2. **Rice:** In a separate pan, boil 2 cups of water and cook 1 cup of wild rice. Set aside once cooked.
3. **Chicken and Broccoli:** Stir-fry garlic and olive oil until garlic is slightly brown. Add chopped uncooked chicken and stir until fully cooked. Add broccoli and top with cover for 3-4 minutes.
4. Mix all 3 together in large bowl.
5. Scoop into separate bowls and serve with mixed green salad. Dress salad with (lemon juice, extra virgin olive oil, sea salt, pinch cayenne pepper, chopped basil or parsley).

Salad Dressings:

Combine one or two from each letter in a blender or bowl :

A: **2 cups of any of the following organic oils:** extra virgin olive oil, Flax, Sunflower, Safflower or Almond.

B: **½ cup of any of the following:** rice vinegar, apple cider, lime, lemon, mustard 1/2 cup

C: 2-3 tbsps. of any of the following: honey, maple syrup, agave

D: **1-2 tbsp. of spices (1-2 or all):** fresh pepper, sea salt, Cayenne pepper, cumin 1-2 tbsp.

E: **1-2 tbsps. Herbs:** rosemary, oregano, dill, mint, garlic, parsley, basil 1-2 tbsp

F: **Veggies:** chopped onions ¼ cup

Blend (to taste) all on low speed in blender or whip with fork in bowl. Save for future use.

Doug's Secret Protein Meal

I love this one for a post workout snack or as a meal.

Ingredients
- 1 lb. ground sautéed free range turkey, chicken or 5-8 scrambled egg whites.
- 1 -2 cups cooked brown rice.
- 1-2 tablespoons organic apricot preserves
- Optional: 1 tbsp. chopped raw nuts (almonds, pistachios or cashews)
- Optional: handful fresh shredded parmesan cheese
- Optional: Trader Joes Green Dragon Hot Sauce to taste
- Optional: 1-2 cups organic steamed or raw chopped veggies (spinach, broccoli, peppers)

Directions
Place all in a bowl and mix well.

Ceviche

Ingredients
- 1 lb. raw fish (cod, shrimp, sea bass fillets, red snapper fillet, mahi mahi, calamari , bay scallops)
- 1 cup diced fresh organic tomato
- tablespoons chopped parsley
- 1/2 teaspoon sea salt
- 1/4 teaspoon pepper
- 2-3 jalapeno peppers, chopped
- 1 medium red onion, finely chopped
- 1 dash hot sauce (your heat liking)
- Lettuce leaf (to line serving bowls)
- ½ cup chopped avocado (optional)
- limes, juiced
- 2 tomatoes, diced

- 5 green onions, minced
- 3 stalks celery, chopped
- 1/2 green bell pepper, minced
- 2 tablespoons extra virgin olive oil
- 1/8 cup chopped fresh cilantro

Directions
1. Rinse your favorite fish (my favorite is the seafood mixture from Trader Joe's : scallops, shrimp and fish and place in a medium sized bowl. Pour lime juice over the fish mixture until completely immersed. Place the mixture in fridge all day or overnight until fish are opaque.
2. Pour out 1/2 of the lime juice and add all veggies, olive oil, sea salt, jalapeno peppers, hot sauce and cilantro to the fish mixture. Stir gently.
3. Eat this for a snack, meal, or whenever you're getting a craving for food.

Chicken Soup

Ingredients:
- 2-16 ounce boxes or cans of Free Range Chicken
- Broth (If you use bouillon cubes loaded with preservatives and salt, then you don't get it. Throw this book out now!)
- 2 chopped Large organic carrots
- 2 cups water
- 2 chopped large celery
- 2 chopped red potatoes
- 1 large white onion
- 4 large bone in chicken breast (no skin)
- Sea salt and pepper
- Cayenne pepper
- 1 clove garlic
- 2 handfuls fresh chopped parsley

Procedure:
1. Boil 2 Cups water and 1 box of chicken broth
2. Place the chicken into boiling water. Once cooked, take out the breast and place into a bowl to cool down and pull the chicken off the bone in small pieces.
3. Place the bones back into the broth along with the chopped onion, celery, garlic, onion and cubed potatoes. Simmer on low for 20 minutes.
4. Add another box of chicken broth and parsley for more 10 minutes.
5. Place chicken back into pot and let cool down for another 9 minutes.
6. Serve over brown rice as is.

No time to make soup? No problem. There are so many tasty, good-for-you soups out there:

Amy's: Lentil (my favorite canned soup)

Whole Foods Prepared: Mom's Chicken Soup, Lentil Soup, Braised Beef or Turkey Chili

Trader Joes: Lentil and 5 grain (refrigerated section). I cut this with 1 cup of water.

FITNESS SHIT

CARDIO:

Guys you've got to do the cardio. Cardio is the most important component besides cardio. There's nothing more satisfying to me than wrestling, fighting or boxing a muscle head who has no muscular endurance. They look so pretty while being thrown on their dome or looking up at the celling.

Benefit of Short/Intensive Cardio Training:
- Burns fat using glycogen (stored sugar)
- Increases Cardio Endurance for short burst activity
- Increases Muscle Fiber i.e. sprinting (FYI; sprinting is great for building your calves, legs and butt
- Burns calories quick

Benefits of Longer/Aerobic Cardo Training:
- Boost capillary density and oxygen transport
- Elevates lung diffusion capacity
- Uses primarily fat for fuel at one hour as long as its challenging and constant level of heart rate elevation
- Great for endorphin elevation (hormones to better your mood)

Summary: apply both types of cardio training to burn fat. Eat less and feel healthier.

Basic Cardio Guide:

Guy 1 and 3:
30 min intense cardio to burn fat (3-4 days week)
90 minutes of cardio to burn calories and deal with stress (2 days week)

Guy 2:
20-30 minutes of intense cardio to burn fat and keep muscle.
(4 days week)

WORKOUTS

Ready to Kick Your Ass Into Shape? You're only as old as your mind tells you. Unless you have a physical ailment that prevents you from your true potential. Either way, get up and kick ass every day!

Pick a workout based on your goal. Commit to one program. If you want to switch personas (business, single or sports guy) once you're done (completing your first program), then go for it.

Just set a goal and complete it. If you don't feel like it's working for you after 3 weeks, then train harder. Don't give up. You have to work for it. Fuck reading pages and a bunch of scientific studies. Train your ass off.

Why should I perform phase 1 first?
I recommend everyone to perform this program first. It will help you increase muscle and cardio endurance.

You will feel great after 3 weeks If you combine both the **PHASE 1 PROGRAM** and **The Bottom Line diet**.

Are these boxing workouts legit?

These workouts are based on real boxing instructional workouts to sweat your ass off and give you the proper foundation to knock out any UFC wannabe (This includes the muscle heads who wear the UFC shirt but have never thrown a punch).

What's the key to make these workouts work?

Intensity and consistency. Train like an athlete with a mission to accomplish your goal. Eat lean, train hard, and go for it. These workouts aren't the bull shit 7 minute or even the jump around douche shit.

What's the best cardio workout?
Run, sprint, box and run. Need I say more? If you can't run. Hit the heavy bag, row, bike or swim.

Why box?
I think you'll find it fun. Relieves stress. Works your entire body. Helps you with agility, stamina and coordination. Most importantly, helps you look athletic and not like a tight ass meat head. Save that look for the teens.

Workout Keys & Tips for Programs:
Reps: Beginner / Advanced (right of forward slash equals the reps for advanced fitness person and left of forward slash equals the reps for a beginner fitness person).

Beginner Fitness: haven't lifted for years or months due to injury or other reason. Just started lifting and are very inconsistent with training.

Advanced Fitness: fit or have lifted for 3 months or longer. Have more time.

Dbs. = dumbbells

Home: or Gym: = perform the certain exercises if you're training at home or the gym. i.e. Gym: Leg press 8 / 8 or Home: Alternate Lunges 15 each leg / 10 each leg. This means if you're at the gym, you'll perform leg press and if at home without a leg press you'll perform lunges.

80% = 80% of max weight (basically 80 -90 percent should be a struggle on your last reps which will be short reps (5-8 reps). Example: you curl 30lbs for max dumbbells. Program says, regular curls, db. 6 reps (90%) = curl 20-25lb dumbbells for 6 reps. Obviously it won't be exact but always remember your workouts should be challenging.

5 reps = heavy and challenging

Gym: = perform if you're in the gym with access to the equipment

5 x 10 = 5 reps x 10 reps (80-90% x 60-80%). This will represent performing an exercise 5 reps @80-90% then dropping to a lower weight 60-80% max to perform 10 reps of the same exercise immediately after the first 5 reps.

Train with intensity for every workout. Shorter workout option is for those with limited time 30 minutes. You must go quickly with no rest at your own risk.

Beginners should always rest when needed and work on form.

Always stretch and warm up.

Repeat 3x = Perform the entire circuit then go back and repeat 3 more times. Total of 4x before proceeding to the next circuit. If you find any of the circuits are too challenging then eliminate a repeat of the circuit. i.e. if the program says, "repeat 3x". Then you should repeat the circuit 1-2x.

WHAT IF I DON'T HAVE ENOUGH TIME TO DO THE WORKOUTS?

Try to make time or perform at least 2-3 sets of each circuit that requires more than 3 sets. Make sure you lift 80-90% max If you can only perform 2-3 sets. For best results, follow the programs as written.

WHAT ARE THE KEYS TO MAKING GAINS!

Lift heavy with intensity. Push every rep with good form. Make sure you're last rep is a struggle. Push yourself to lift heavier weights with every workout and/or every week. If you're a beginner, lift very slowly and don't over train. Your first few weeks should be more about keeping good form, higher reps and keeping the weights @60-80 % max weights to get your tendons and muscles ready for higher weights. Refuel after every workout with good nutrition.

KEYS TO LESS INJURY!

Progress slowly. Drink water everyday at least ½ gallon per day. Stretch after a warm up (10 – 15 minute warm up with lighter sets and/or cardio).

LIFTING QUESTIONS YOU MAY HAVE:

Can I get big with lighter weights and less reps?

Sure, you can develop muscle with lighter weights and strict form. Simply, you just have to exaggerate the contraction while lifting and go down slower when performing a negative contraction (i.e. lowering a straight bar when curling). However, you won't get stronger after a certain period of time and you're muscle density won't be that of someone who lifts heavier. I.e. the difference in physique of someone who does cross fit or someone who is a body builder.

What if I'm very skinny and I just can't put on size?

You'll have to concentrate on heavier lifts, high calorie meals and less cardio. You should be eating at least 5 meals a day made up of complex carbs 50%, lean proteins 30%, omega-3 fats 20%.

Why do you have boxing integrated into the workouts?

Boxing workouts are great to burn fat, learn self-defense and train your entire body all at the same time. Simply performing just burpees, mountain climbers and jumping jacks is copy-cat shit (amateur training). Plus, nothing is worse than a guy who's jacked and looks tough but in reality is a big pussy. Does that answer your question? Note: just hitting a bag and performing a perfect jab, cross doesn't make you tough either. However, it's better than not knowing how to punch.

Will cardio hinder my muscle growth?

Yes and no. If you're looking to put on 50 lbs. You should avoid cardio sessions over 15 minutes in duration. However, you can attain muscle mass while integrating cardio sessions into your program as long as you're eating the proper nutrition, resting, training with intensity, lifting heavy and taking in more calories than you're burning. Long duration cardio sessions, 90 minutes and greater, may break down your muscle tissue. Again, this book is to help you get muscular and fit. You should use different programs, if you're trying to just be a meat head.

What if these workouts are too long?

Lift heavy, eliminate 1 or 2 of the circuits and train balls to the walls. Go, go and go. Pyramiding the weights is fine for every set. Hence, if you can only do 3 sets of bench rather than 5. On the 3rd set perform 2-4 reps 95 percent then drop down to 80% for another 4-5 reps then perform as many reps as you can @60%.

READY TO START TRAINING?

I have created workouts for all 3 guys. Make sure to pick the workout that fits your profile. Each workout consist of 2 phases. I suggest everyone perform phase 1 whether your goals is to pack on muscle or just to get fit. Phase 1 will get you ready to make more gains with Phase 2.

PHASE 1 (ALL GUYS)

SUGGESTED FOR ALL GUYS FOR THE FIRST 21 DAYS

I highly recommend everyone do this workout program first to bring up your cardio to another level, build muscular endurance, knock off fat and get fit. This phase will definitely help change your body. Even if you feel like you're fit. Start with this program first.

KEY:
BEGINNER REPS / ADVANCED REPS

Week 1

DAY 1

CIRCUIT 1
1. Jump Rope 1 min / 2 min
2. Push Ups 5-15 / 25-50
3. *Battle rope, alternate 30 sec / 1 min

Repeat all 3, Beginner: 5-8 x / Advanced: 4-5 x
*No battle rope? Perform jumping jacks with 1-2 lbs. weights in each hand.

CIRCUIT 2
1. Mountain Climbers 30 sec / 1 min
2. Jumping squats 5-10 / 10 w 20 lb. medicine ball

Repeat both, beginner: 10x / Advanced: 10x

CARDIO
Jog:
Beginner: 15 min / Advanced: 20-45 min

DAY 2

CIRCUIT 1:
1. Tricep Push Ups 5 / 10
2. Sit Ups 5 / 10
3. Leg Lifts 10 / 25

Repeat all 3, no rest if possible,
Beginner: 1-3 minutes / Advanced: 2-3 minutes

CIRCUIT 2:
1. Jump Rope 1 min / 1 min
2. Boxing Level 1 (foot work) 3 min / 3 min

Repeat both no rest if possible,
Beginner: 2-4 x / Advanced: 3-5 x

*Boxing Level 1 (Foot Work):
Stepping Forward To Back, Back To Front 1 min
Stepping Right To Left, Left To Right 1 min
Open Leg Shuffle Right and Left 1 min

CARDIO
Jog:
Beginner: 10 min / Advanced: 15 min plus sprints below

Advanced Only:
Stretch hamstrings, lower back and quads 5 min
  • Sprints 5 x 25 yards, walk back for rest

*Boxing Video Workouts

For Demo Video of all boxing workouts Subscribe at www.fitactions.com/builditworkoutvideos

DAY 3

CIRCUIT 1
1. Jump Rope 1 min / 2 min
2. Shoulder Press Dumbbell or Bar 10 (50-70%) / 15 (70-80%)

Repeat both, no rest if possible,
Beginner: 2-3 x / Advanced: 3-4 x

CIRCUIT 2
1. Battle Rope (rope slams) 1 min / 2 min
2. Shoulder: Front To Side Raises 5 reps (50-70%) / 5 reps (70-90%)
3. Upright Rows (db or bar) 10 reps (70-80%) / 8-12 reps (80-90%)

Repeat all 3, no rest if possible,
Beginner: 2-3 x / Advanced: 3-4 x

CIRCUIT 3
1. ABS: bicycle 30 sec / 30 sec min
2. ABS: Knee Tucks 5-10 / 15-25
3. ABS: Plank, Forearms 30 sec / 30 sec
4. ABS: High Plank, Hands 30 sec / 30 sec
5. ABS: Hanging Leg Raises, Skip / 30 sec

Repeat all 4 - 5, no rest if possible
Beginner: 1-3x / Advanced: 3-5 x

CARDIO
JOG:
Beginner: 15 min / Advanced: 20 – 30 minutes

DAY 4

CIRCUIT 1
1. Jumping Jacks 10
2. Squat 10
3. Jumping Squat 10
4. Stand Ups 5 each leg (see leg exercises)

Repeat all 4, no rest if possible
Beginner: 1-2 min / Advanced: 3-5 min

CIRCUIT 2
1. Flat Bench Press, dumbbells 10 reps (50-60%) / 10 reps (70-80%)
2. Squats with Bar or Dumbbell 10 reps (50%) / 12-15 reps (70-80%)
3. If at Home: *Alternate Lunges 10 reps each side (50%) / 10 reps each side (70%) or If at the gym: Leg Press 15 reps (60%) / 15 reps (70-80%).

*Lunges: hold dumbbells on each side.
Repeat all 3, No rest if possible,
Beginner: 1-3 x / Advanced: 3-4 x

CIRCUIT 3
*Boxing Level 1 (Basic Punches)
Repeat All punches 10x (100 reps of each punch)

CARDIO
Jog
Beginner: 10-15 min (pick up pace) / Advanced: 10-15 min

Advanced Only:

Sprints (stretch legs, lower back and upper back)

- 5 x 25 yards, rest with a walk back
- 5 x 50 yards, rest with a walk back
- 1 x 100 yards, rest with a walk back

*Boxing Video Workouts

For Demo Video of all boxing workouts Subscribe at www.fitactions.com/builditworkoutvideos

DAY 5

CARDIO

Jog

Beginner: 30 Min / Advanced: 30-45 min

Circuit 1

1. Straight Bar or Dumbbell Curls 12 reps (50-70%) / 12 (70-90%)
2. Push Ups 10 reps / 25-50
3. *Power Pull Ups 30 sec / 30 sec

*Your feet should be on ground or low-profile box while you hang from the bar. Arms locked out, jump and pull at the same time. The Jump should assist you but not do all the work. Once at top pause with chin over bar 2 long sec and hop down while still holding bar. Immediately explode back up and repeat entire time noted in program. Try to let your down with some resistance.

Tricep Dips (TD) or Dips (D) : TD 20-30 D 3-10 / TD 30-50 D 5-20

Repeat all 4, No rest if possible,

Beginner: 1-3 x / Advanced 3-4 x

DAY 6

Boxing Level 1 (Foot Work)
Beginner: 3 min / Advanced: 3 min

Boxing Level 1 (Basic Punches)
Beginner and Advanced: Repeat all 10x

CIRCUIT 1
1. Shoulder Press bar or db   6 (70-80%) / 6 (80-90%)
2. Bent Over Raises   8 (60-70%) / 8 (70-80%)
3. Upright Rows   6 (60-70%) / 6 (80-90%)
4. Battle Rope (alternate arms sitting) 30 sec / 1 min

Repeat all 4, No rest if possible,
Beginner: 2-3 x/ Advanced 3-5 X

CIRCUIT 2
1. Squats Bar or goblet Db 6 (70-80%) / 6 (80-90%)
2. Home (lunges) 10 each side / 10 each side holding 10-20lbs **or** if at the Gym (leg press) 12 (70%) / 15 (80%)
3. Home (back leg ball curls) 15 / 25 **or** if at the Gym (back leg curls) 10 (50%) / 10-15 (70-90%)
4. Sit Ups 25 / 50
5. Leg Raises 10 / 25
6. Kickouts 5-10 / 10-30

Repeat all 6, No rest if Possible,
Beginner 2-3x, Advanced 4-5x

CARDIO
Beginner and Advanced: Jog 1-2 miles or Bike 20 min

DAY 7

Stretch and Rest
Or
Stretch and Cardio 30-90 min

WEEK 2

DAY 8

CIRCUIT 1
1. 1 Jump Rope 1 min / 2 min
2. 2 Elevated Push Ups 5-15 / 25-50
3. 3 Sit Up w Cross, Cross 5-10 / 25-50

Repeat all 3, Beginner: 3-6 x / Advanced: 3-5 x

CIRCUIT 2
1. Mountain Climbers 30 sec / 1 min
2. Jumping squats 5-10 reps / 10 reps w 20 lb. medicine ball
3. Back N' Forth (see cardio exercises) 30 sec / 1 min

Repeat all 3, beginner: 3-5 x / Advanced: 5- 10 x

CARDIO
Jog:
Beginner: 15-20 min / Advanced: 20-45 min

DAY 9

CIRCUIT 1:
1. Push Ups 5 / 25-50
2. Sit Ups w twist 5 / 25
3. Hanging knee raises or Knee Tucks 10 / 25

4. 45 Degree Crunches 15 sec / 30 sec
5. Bicycle 30 sec / 1 min

Repeat all 5, no rest if possible,
Beginner: 2-3 x / Advanced: 2-4 x

CIRCUIT 2:
1. Jump Rope 1 min / 1 min
2. Boxing Level 1 (foot work) 3 min / 3 min
3. Fast High Knee Run 1 min / 1 min

Repeat all 3, no rest if possible,
Beginner: 1-2 x / Advanced: 2-3 x

*Boxing Level 1 (Foot Work):
Stepping Forward To Back, Back To Front 1.5 min
Stepping Right To Left, Left To Right 1.5 min

CARDIO
Jog:
Beginner: 10 min / Advanced: 15 min plus sprints below
Advanced Only:
Stretch hamstrings, lower back and quads
Sprints:
5 x 25 yards, walk back for rest
5 x 50 yards, walk back for rest
1: 300 (start at zero line, sprint to 50, touch line, turn and sprint back to zero line, touch line, sprint back to 50 and so on. You'll repeat sprinting to 50 line and from 50 yard line to zero, 3x total. Hence, the 300. No rest and full sprint.
Can't Sprint Outside? Treadmill: 10-15 min jog with 30 sec sprints every other minute. Note: not as effective as outside running.

*Boxing Video Workouts
For Demo Video of all boxing workouts Subscribe at

www.fitactions.com/builditworkoutvideos

DAY 10

CIRCUIT 1
1. Jump Rope 1 min / 2 min
2. Shoulder Press Dumbbell or Bar 10 (50-60%) / 10-12 (70-80%)
3. Bent Over Raises 10 (50-60%) / 8-12 (70-80%)

Repeat all 3, no rest if possible,
Beginner: 2-4 x / Advanced: 3-5 x

CIRCUIT 2
1. Battle Rope (alternate arms) 1 min / 2 min
2. Shoulder Raises Side to 45 degrees to Front Raises 6 reps (50%) / 6 reps (60-70%)
3. Upright Rows (db or bar) 10 reps (60-70%) / 8-12 reps (70-90%)
4. Shrugs 15 reps (70-80%) / 12-15 reps (80-90%)

Repeat all 4, no rest if possible,
Beginner: 2-3 x / Advanced: 3–5 x

CIRCUIT 3
1. *Power Pull Ups 30 sec / 30 sec – 1 min
2. Power (clapping) Push Ups (knees) 30 sec / 30 sec – 1 min
3. Jump Rope (high knee running or skip) 1 min / 2 min

Power Pull Ups: Your feet should be on ground or low-profile box while you hang from the bar. Arms locked out, jump and pull at the same time. The Jump should assist you but not do all the work. Once at top pause with chin over bar 2 long sec and hop down while still holding bar. Immediately explode back up and repeat entire time noted in program. Try to let your down with some resistance.

Repeat all 3, no rest if possible

Beginner: 2-3 x, Advanced: 3-5 x

CARDIO
JOG:
Beginner: 15 min / Advanced 15 – 30 minutes

DAY 11

CIRCUIT 1
1. Jumping Jacks 10
2. Squat w medicine ball 10 (10lb) / 10 (20lb)
3. Jumping Squat 10 / 10

Repeat all, no rest if possible
Beginner: 2 min / Advanced: 3-5 min

CIRCUIT 2
1. Flat Bench Press or on fitness ball, dumbbells 6 reps (70-80%) / 5 reps (90-95%)
2. Incline Bench Press or on fitness ball, dumbbells 6 rep (80-90%) / 6 reps (80-90%)
3. Squats with Bar or Dumbbell 10 reps (70%) / 10 reps (80%)
4. **If at Home** (Alternate Lunges) 10 reps (hold 10lbs each arm) /10 reps (15-20lbs each arm) or **if at Gym** (leg press): 8 reps (80%) / 8-12 reps (80-90%)

Repeat all 4, No rest if possible,
Beginner: 2-4 x / Advanced: 4 - 6 x

CIRCUIT 3
*Boxing Level 1 (Basic Punches)
Perform all Punches, No rest if possible, 10x (100 each punch)

CARDIO
Jog

Beginner: 10-15 min (pick up pace) / Advanced: 10-15 min
Advanced Only:
Sprints (stretch legs, lower back and upper back)
- 5 x 25 yards, rest with a walk back
- 5 x 50 yards, rest with a walk back
- 5 x 100 yards, rest with a jog back

*Boxing Video Workouts
For Demo Video of all boxing workouts Subscribe at www.fitactions.com/builditworkoutvideos

DAY 12

CARDIO
Jog
Beginner: 30 Min / Advanced: 30-45 min

Circuit 1
1. Band Curls 30 sec fast / 1 min fast
2. Tricep Push Ups 10 / 10-20
3. Straight Bar or Dumbbell Curls12 (50-70%) / 12 (60-70%)
4. *Power CHIN Ups 30 sec / 1min
5. Concentration Curls 10 each arm / 10 each arm

*Power CHIN ups: Your feet should be on ground or low-profile box while you hang from the bar. Arms locked out, jump and pull at the same time. The Jump should assist you but not do all the work. Once at top pause with chin over bar 2 long sec and hop down while still holding bar. Immediately explode back up and repeat entire time noted in program. Try to let your down with some resistance.

6. Tricep Dips Bench (TDB) or Dips (D)
7. TDB 20-30 D 3-10 / TDB 30-50 D 5-20

Repeat all 6, No rest if possible,

Beginner: 2-4 x / Advanced 3-5 x

DAY 13

Boxing Level 1 (Foot Work)
Beginner: 3 min / Advanced: 3 min

Boxing Level 1 (Basic Punches)
Beginner and Advanced: Repeat all Punches 10x

Boxing Level 1 (Bag 1)
Beginner: 3 min / Advanced: 3 min

CIRCUIT 1
1. Shoulder Press bar or db 6 (60-80%) / 6 (80-90%)
2. Bent Over Raises 8 (50-60%) / 8 (60-80%)
3. Upright Rows 6 (70-80%) / 6 (80-90%)
4. Battle Rope (alternate arms sitting) 30 sec / 1 min

Repeat all 4, No rest if possible,
Beginner: 2-3 x / Advanced 4- 5 X

CIRCUIT 2
1. Squats Bar or Db 6 (70%) / 6 (80-90%)
2. Stand Ups 10 each leg / 25 each leg
3. Jumping Squats 10 no mb / 10 with medicine ball (20-30lb)
4. **If at Home (back leg ball curls):** 15 / 25 or **If at Gym** (back leg curls): 10 (50-60%) / 10-15 (70-80%)
5. Sit Ups 25 / 50

Repeat all 5, No rest if Possible,
Beginner 2-3 x / Advanced 4-5 x

CIRCUIT 3

CARDIO
Jog
Beginner and Advanced: 1-3 miles or Bike 20 min

DAY 14

Stretch and Rest
Or
Stretch and Cardio 30-90 min

DAY 15

CIRCUIT 1
1. Jump Rope 1 min / 2 min
2. Push Ups 5-15 / 25-50
3. Sit Up w Cross, Cross 5-10 /25-50
4. Pull Ups 30 sec / 30 sec

Repeat all 4, Beginner: 3-5 x / Advanced: 4-5 x

CIRCUIT 2
1. Skating 30 sec / 1 min
2. Jumping squats 5-10 / 10 w/ 20 lb. medicine ball
3. Back N Forth 30 sec / 1 min
4. Mountain Climbers 30 sec / 1 min

Repeat all 4, beginner: 8 x / Advanced: 8 x

CARDIO
Jog:
Beginner: 10 min / Advanced: 20-30 min

DAY 16

CIRCUIT 1:
1. Elevated Push Ups 5 / 10
2. Sit Ups w/ Cross, Cross 5 / 10
3. Leg Lifts 10 / 20
4. Hanging Leg Raises or Knee Tucks 10 / 20

Repeat all 4, no rest if possible,
Beginner: 3-5 minutes / Advanced: 5-10 minutes

CIRCUIT 2:
1. Jump Rope 1 min / 1 min
2. *Boxing Level 1 (Foot Work) 3 min / 3 min
3. Run High Knee 1 min / 1 min
4. Star Jumps 10 / 25

Repeat all 4, no rest if possible,
Beginner: 3-4 x / Advanced: 4-5 x

*Boxing Level 1 (Foot Work):
Stepping Forward To Back, Back To Front 1.5 min
Stepping Right To Left, Left To Right 1.5 min

CARDIO
Jog:
Beginner: 15 min / Advanced: 15-20 min plus below

Advanced Only:
Stretch hamstrings, lower back and quads
Sprints:
5 x 25 yards, walk back for rest
5 x 50 yards, walk back for rest
3: 300 (start at zero line, sprint to 50, touch line, turn and sprint back to zero line, touch line, sprint back to 50 and so on. You'll repeat

sprinting to 50 line and back to start 3x total. Hence, the 300. No rest and full sprint. If you can only sprint at an area that allows 25 yards then do the same 6x.

Can't Sprint Outside? Treadmill: 15 min jog (jog for a minute and sprint 30 sec sprints every other minute for the entire 15 minutes.) Note: not as effective as outside running.

*Boxing Video Workouts

For Demo Video of all boxing workouts Subscribe at www.fitactions.com/builditworkoutvideos

DAY 17

CIRCUIT 1
1. Jump Rope 1 min / 2 min
2. Shoulder Press Dumbbell or Bar 10 reps (70-80%) / 8-10 reps (80-90%)
3. Bent Over Raises 10 rep (60-70%) / 8-12 reps (70-90%)
4. Power Pull Ups 30 sec / 1 min

Repeat all 4, no rest if possible,
Beginner: 3-4 x / Advanced: 4-5 x

CIRCUIT 2
1. Battle Rope (Double arm slam) 30 reps / 50 reps
2. Shoulder Raises: Side to 45 degrees to Front raises 5 reps (80%) / 5 reps (80-90%)
3. Upright Rows (db or bar) 5 reps (90% max) / 5 reps (90% max)
4. Upright Rows (db or bar) till failure,(80% max) / till failure (80%)
5. Shrugs 10-12 reps (80-90%) / 15 reps (80-90%)

Repeat all 5, no rest if possible,
Beginner: 2-3 x / Advanced: 4-5 x

CIRCUIT 3
1. ABS: bicycle 30 sec / 30 sec
2. ABS: Knee Tucks 5-10 / 20-30
3. ABS: Plank, Forearms or ball 30 sec / 1 min
4. ABS: Plank, Hands 30 sec / 30 sec
5. ABS: Leg Lifts 10 / 20
6. Power (clapping) Push Ups (knees) 10 / 20-30

Repeat all 6, no rest if possible
Beginner: 2-3 x, Advanced: 4-5 x

CARDIO
JOG:
Beginner: 15 min / Advanced: 15 – 30 minutes

DAY 18

CIRCUIT 1
1. Jumping Jacks 10
2. Squat w medicine ball 10 reps (10lb) / 10 reps (20lb)
3. Jumping Squat 10 reps (10lb) / 10 reps (20lb)
4. Stand Ups with medicine ball 5 each leg / 10 each leg

Repeat all, no rest if possible
Beginner: 5 min / Advanced: 5-10 min

CIRCUIT 2
1. Flat Bench Press or on fitness ball, dumbbells 5 reps (15-35 lbs.) / 5 reps (35-80lbs)
2. Incline Bench Press or on fitness ball, dumbbells 6 reps (15-35 lbs.) / 6 reps (35-80 lbs.)
3. Overhead Pulls db. 10 reps (70%) /10-15 reps (80-90%)
4. Squats with Bar or Goblet Dumbbell 8 reps (60-70%) / 8 reps (80-90%)

5. **If at Home** (Alternate Lunges):15 reps w dbs. (10-15lbs) / 10 reps (15-25lbs each arm) **or if at the Gym** (Leg Press): 12 reps (80-90%) / drop set: 10 reps (90%) x 10 reps (80%) x 10 reps (60-70%)

Repeat all 5, No rest if possible,
Beginner: 2-4x / Advanced: 3-5 x

CIRCUIT 3
*Boxing Level 1 (Basic Punches)
Perform all Punches. No rest if possible
Repeat All punches 10x (100 each punch)

CARDIO
Jog

Beginner: 10-15 min (pick up pace) / Advanced: 10-15 min

SPRINTS:
Beginner:
Sprints 5 x 10 yards, rest with a walk back
Sprints 4 x 25 yards, rest with a walk back

Advanced Only:
Sprints (stretch legs, lower back and upper back)
- 5 x 25 yards, rest with a walk back
- 5 x 50 yards, rest with a walk back
- 5 x 100 yards, rest with a jog back
- Sprint 10 yards, turn, drop for 5 push-ups, turn sprint 10 yards and repeat till failure.

*Boxing Video Workouts
For Demo Video of all boxing workouts Subscribe at www.fitactions.com/builditworkoutvideos

DAY 19

CARDIO
Jog
Beginner: 30 Min / Advanced: 30 min

Circuit 1
1. Straight Bar or Dumbbell Curls 5 reps (80-90% max) / 5 (80-90% max)
2. Straight Bar or Dumbbell Curls10 reps (70-80%) /10-till failure (70-80%)
3. Band Curls 30 sec fast / 1 min fast
4. Push Ups 10 reps / 10-20 reps
5. * Power Pull Ups 30 sec / 1min
6. Concentration Curls 10 reps each arm (70%) / 5 reps each arm (90%)
7. Concentration Curls, Advanced only: till failure each arm (70-80%)

* Pull ups: Your feet should be on ground or low-profile box while you hang from the bar. Arms locked out, jump and pull at the same time. The Jump should assist you but not do all the work. Once at top pause with chin over bar 2 long sec and hop down while still holding bar. Immediately explode back up and repeat entire time noted in program. Try to let your down with some resistance.

8. Tricep Dips Bench (TBD) or Dips (D)
9. TDB 20-30 D 3-10 / TDB 30-50 D 5-20

Repeat all 8, No rest if possible,
Beginner: 2-4x / Advanced 4-6x

DAY 20

CIRCUIT 1
1. Shoulder Press (bar or dbs.) 6 reps (90%)/ 6 reps (90%)
2. Bent Over Raises 8 reps (70%) / 8 reps (80-90%)
3. Upright Rows 6 reps (80%) / 6 reps (90%)
4. Battle Rope (alternate arms sitting) 30 sec / 1 min

Repeat all 4, No rest if possible,
Beginner: 2-3 x / Advanced 4-6 X

CIRCUIT 2
1. Squats Bar or Goblet Db 6 reps (80-90%) / 6 reps (80-90%)
2. Jumping Squats 10 reps (5-10lb *mb) / 10 reps (20lb mb)
3. If at Home (ball curls) 15/ 25 or Gym (Back Leg Curls): 10 (70%) / 10-15 (80%-90%)
4. Sit Ups 25 reps / 50 reps

Repeat all 4, No rest if Possible,
Beginner 2-3x / Advanced 4-5x

*mb = medicine ball

Boxing Level 1 (Foot Work)
Beginner: 3 min / Advanced: 3 min

Boxing Level 1 (Basic Punches)
Beginner and Advanced: Repeat all Punches 10x

Boxing Level 1 (Bag 1)
Beginner: 2 x 3 min / Advanced: 3 x 3 min
Rest 30 sec – 1 min between rounds

*Boxing Video Workouts
For Demo Video of all boxing workouts Subscribe at www.fitactions.com/builditworkoutvideos

DAY 21

Rest and Stretch
Or
Stretch and Cardio: 30-90 minutes

Well that's Phase 1. Ready to start Phase 2?
I need you to pick which guy fits your profile (Business Guy, Single Guy or Sports Guy). Follow these plans as close as possible.
See Below for all plans:

BUSINESS GUY
I'm giving you 2 workout options (quick or longer workout) for each day. I realize every day brings challenges to get a workout in. Obviously, the longer workouts will give you better results. However, the shorter workouts still work if you stick to the diet I showed in this book. The shorter workouts are very challenging. The key: to use heavier weights, very little rest if any, and train with intensity.
If any workout is too long or your short on time. Don't skip a workout if possible. Simply, perform only 2 sets of each circuit.

PHASE 2

DAY 1

OPTION 1 (QUICK WORKOUT)
Warm Up
1. Jumping Jacks 30 sec
2. High Knee Running 30 sec
3. Tricep Push Ups 15 sec
4. Push Ups 15 sec
5. Sit Ups 30 sec

Repeat all 5 exercises, 4x

CIRCUIT 1:
1. Flat Chest Press (fitness ball or bench) 5 reps (70%) / 5 reps (90%)
2. Incline Chest Press (fitness ball or bench) 10 reps (70%) / 8 reps (80%)
3. Flat Flies (fitness ball or bench) 10 reps / *5 reps x 5 reps (90% x 80%)

*Drop set Heavy for 5 reps to Lighter weight for 5 reps
Repeat all 3, no rest if possible
Beginner: 1-3 x / Advanced: 3-4 x

CIRCUIT 2:
1. Jump Rope 1 min / 1 min

2. Squats Bar or Dumbbell 10 reps (70% max) / 20 reps (60-70% max)
3. *Battle Rope, alternate 30 sec / 1 min
*No rope? Throw Straight Punches in air with 1-2 lbs. for same time

Repeat all 3 exercises, no rest if possible
Beginner: 1-3 x / Advanced: 3-4 x

OPTION 2 (LONGER WORKOUT)
Warm Up
1. Jumping Jacks 30 sec
2. High Knee Running 30 sec
3. Power Push Ups 15 sec
4. Push Ups 15 sec
5. Crunches 30 sec

Repeat all 5 exercises, 4x

CIRCUIT 1:
1. Flat Chest Press, dbs. (fitness ball or bench) 5 reps (70%) / 5 reps (90%)
2. Incline Chest Press (fitness ball or bench) 10 reps (70%) / 8 reps (80%)
3. Flat Flies, dbs. (fitness ball or bench) 10 reps / *5 x 5 reps (90% x 80%)
4. Overhead pulls 10 reps (70% max) / *5 x 10 reps (90% x 80%)
5. Shrugs 6 reps (80%) / 8-10 reps (80%)
*Drop set: Heavy to Lighter weight

Repeat all 5, no rest if possible
Beginner: 1-3 x / Advanced: 3-5 x

CIRCUIT 2:
1. Jump Rope 1 min / 1 min
2. Squats Bar or DB 10 reps (70% max) / 20 reps (70% max)

3. Jumping Squats 10 reps (5-10lb *mb) / 10 reps (15-25lb mb)
4. **Battle Rope, rope slams 30 sec / 1 min

*Mb = medicine ball

**No rope? Throw Straight Punches in air with 1-2 lbs. for same time

Repeat all 4, no rest if possible
Beginner: 1-3 x / Advanced: 3-5 x

CARDIO:
Jog:
Beginner 1 mile / Advanced: 2-4 miles

DAY 2

OPTION 1 (QUICK WORKOUT)

Boxing Level 1 (Bag) 5 x 3 min rounds
Rest 30 sec – 1 min between rounds

No bag? Throw combinations 2-4 punches, move and repeat with or without 1-2lb. dumbbells

Circuit 2:
1. Jump Rope 1 min
2. Plank 30 sec / 1 min
3. Knee Tucks 30 sec / 1 min
4. Bicycle 30 sec / 30 sec
5. 45 degree Crunches 15 sec / 30 sec
6. Sit Ups 10 / 25

Repeat all 6, no rest if possible
Beginner 1-3 x / Advanced 3-5 x

OPTION 2 (LONGER WORKOUT)

CIRCUIT 1
1. Boxing Level 1 (Bag) Repeat 5 x 3 minute rounds.
    Rest 1 minute or Perform Active Rest In between rounds
    *perform the following 2-3x below:
    1. Push Ups 10
    2. Mountain Climbers 30 sec
    3. Air Squats No Weight 10 reps

*Once you perform all 3 exercises 2-3x, proceed back to boxing level 1 (bag) for a total of 5x.
No bag? Throw 2-4 punch combinations, move and repeat with or without 1-2lb. dumbbells.

Combination examples:
Left Jab, Straight Right, Left Hook
Left Jab, Left Jab, Straight Right
Left Jab, Straight Right, Left Hook, Straight Right
Left Jab, Right Upper Cut, Left Hook, Straight Right

2. Boxing Level 1 (foot Work) 3 min / 3 min

CIRCUIT 2:
1. Jump Rope 1 min / 2 min
2. Plank 30 sec / 1 min
3. Knee Tucks 30 sec / 1 min
4. Bicycle 30 sec / 30 sec
5. 45 degree Crunches 15 sec / 30 sec
6. Sit Ups 10 / 25
7. Hanging leg raises 10 / 30

Repeat all 6, no rest if possible
Beginner 1-3 x / Advanced 3-5 x

DAY 3

OPTION 1 (QUICK WORKOUT)

CIRCUIT 1

1. Jump Rope 1 min
2. Straight Bar Curls 10 reps (60-70%) / 5 reps x 5 reps (90 x 80%)
3. Close Grip Press Triceps 8-10 reps (70-80%) / 8-10 reps (80-90%)
4. Standing Db Curls (same time) 5 reps (80%) / 5 reps (80-90%)
5. Standing Db Curls (alternate) 5 reps (70-80%) / 5-10 reps (70-80%)
6. **If at Gym:** Tricep Rope Push Downs 10 reps (70-80%) / 10 reps (80-90%) **or if at Home:** Dips till failure / till failure

Repeat all 6, no rest if possible
Beginner: 2-3 x / Advanced: 3-4 x

CIRCUIT 2

1. One Arm Row 10 reps (60-70%) / 10 reps (70-90%)
2. Pull Ups till failure / till failure
3. Chin Up till failure / till failure
4. Chin Up – Hold till failure / till failure
5. Shoulder Press Bar 10 reps (50-60%) / 5 reps (80-90%)
6. Shoulder press Dbs (advanced only) 10 reps (70-80%)

Repeat all 5-6, no rest if possible
Beginner: 2-3 x / Advanced: 3-4 x

OPTION 2 (LONGER WORKOUT)

CIRCUIT 1

1. Jump Rope 1 min
2. Straight Bar Curls 10 reps (60-70%) / drop set: 5 reps x 5 reps (90 x 80%)

3. Close Grip Press Triceps 10 reps (70-80%) / 10 reps (80-90%)
4. Standing Db Curls (same time) 5 reps (80%) / 5 reps (80-90%)
5. Standing Db Curls (alternate) 5 reps (70-80%) / 5-10 reps (70-80%)
6. **Gym:** Tricep Rope Push Downs 10 reps (70-80%) / 10-15 reps (80-90%) **or if at Home**: Dips till failure / till failure

Repeat all 6, no rest if possible
Beginner: 2-3x / Advanced: 3- 4 x

CIRCUIT 2
1. One Arm Row 10-12 reps (60-70%) / 10-15 reps (70-90%)
2. Pull Ups till failure / till failure
3. Chin Up till failure / till failure
4. Chin Up – Hold on top (chin over bar) till failure / till failure
5. Shoulder Press Bar 10 reps (50-60%) / 5 reps (80-90%)
6. Shoulder Press Dbs (advanced only) 10 reps (70%)
7. **Gym:** Low Row 8-12 reps (60-70%) / 8-12 reps (70-80%) **or if at Home:** Bent Over Raises 8-12 reps (50-60%) / 8-12 reps (60-70%)
8. Upright Rows dbs 10-12 reps (50-70%) / 10-12 reps (80-90%)

Repeat all 8, no rest if possible
Beginner: 1-3 x / Advanced: 3-4 x

Cardio:

Beginner
Jog 1 mile

Sprints:
5 x 25 yards (rest with a walk back)

Can't run outside? Run on treadmill 12 minutes with sprint 30 sec every other minute.

Advanced:
Jog 1 mile
Sprints:
5 x 25 yards
5 x 50 yards
3 x 100 yards

Can't run outside? Run on treadmill 20 minutes with sprint 1 min every other minute.

DAY 4

OPTION 1 (QUICK WORKOUT)

CIRCUIT 1:
1. Flat Press, dbs. Bench 5 reps (80%) / 5 reps (90%)
2. Incline Press, dbs. Bench 5 reps (80-90%) / 5 reps (90%)
3. Incline Flies, dbs. 15 (60-70%) / 5 x 10 (90 x 60-70%)
4. Shrugs 12-15 reps (50%) / 4-6 reps x 12 reps (90 x 70-80%)

Repeat all 4, no rest if possible
Beginner: 1-3 x / Advanced: 3- 4x

CIRCUIT 2
1. Squats dumbbell or Bar 12 reps (70%) / 12 reps (80%)
2. **If at Gym:** Leg Press (gym) 10 reps (50%) / 15 reps (70%) **Or if at home:** Alternate Lunges 10 each side (hold 10 lbs. each hand) / 15 reps each side (hold 10-20 lbs. each hand)
3. **If at Gym:** Leg Extension 25 reps (50%) / 25 reps (60**%) or if at Home:** Bench Step Ups 15 each leg /10 each leg holding 10-20 lbs. each hand
4. Hanging leg raises 20 reps / 20 reps
5. Sit Ups 10 reps / 25 reps
6. Plank 1 min / 1 min
7. Push Ups 10 reps / 20-50 reps

Repeat all 7, no rest if possible
Beginner: 1-3 x / Advanced: 2-4 x

CIRCUIT 3
1. Punches: left, Right (punch over eye level)- Fast 1 min / 1 min
2. Mountain climbers 1 min / 1 min
3. Punches: hooks to head - Fast 1 min / 1 min
4. Jumping Jacks 1 min / 1min
5. Punches: Upper Cuts to Head - Fast 1 min / 1 min
*all punches in the air

Repeat all 5, no rest if possible
Beginner: 1-2 x / Advanced: 2 x

OPTION 2 (LONGER WORKOUT)

CIRCUIT 1:
1. Flat Press, dbs. Bench or *Fitness Ball 5 reps (80%) / 5 reps (90%)
2. Incline Press, dbs. Bench or Fitness Ball 5 reps (80-90%) / 5 reps (90%)
3. Incline Flies, dbs. 15 reps (70%) / 15 reps (70-80%)
4. **If at Home:** Flat Flies: *5 reps x 10 reps (80 x 70%) / 5 reps x 10 reps (90% x 80%) **or if at the Gym:** Cable Flies drop set: 5 reps x 10 reps (80% x 70%) / 5 reps x 10 reps (90% x 80%)
* drop sets. Start with heaviest weight and drop down every 5 reps. You should be struggling with each set of 5 reps.
* If you don't have a bench use a fitness ball. Make sure you slide down to keep head rested on ball. Flat press: lift hips up by pressing off heels. Incline Press: slide down so your hips drop down and knees bent as you should be at a 45 degree angle on ball with head resting at all times.

Repeat all 4, no rest if possible
Beginner: 1-3 x, Advanced: 2-4 x

CIRCUIT 2
1. Squats dumbbell or Bar 12 reps (70%) / 12 reps (80%)
2. Leg Press (feet straight) 10 reps (50%) / drop set: 15 reps x 10 reps (80% x 70%)
3. Leg Extension (gym) 25 reps (50%) / 25 reps (50-60%)
4. Hanging leg raises 20 / 20
5. Leg Lifts (abs) 1 min / 1 min
6. Sit Ups 10-20 / 25 – 50
7. Kick Outs:abs 10-20 / 20-30
8. Push Ups 10 / 10

Repeat all 8, no rest if possible
Beginner: 2-3 x / Advanced: 2-4 x

CIRCUIT 3
1. Punches: left, Right over eye level - Fast 1 min / 1 min
2. Mountain climbers 1 min / 1 min
3. Punches: hooks to head - Fast 1 min / 1min
4. Jumping Jacks 1 min / 1min
5. Punches: Upper Cuts to Head - Fast 1 min / 1 min
6. Run High Knee 1 min / 1 min
7. 2 straights, 2 hooks, 2 upper cuts 1 min / 2 min

Repeat all 7, no rest if possible
Beginner: 1-2 x / Advanced: 2 x

CARDIO
1. Burpees or Star Jumps 10 reps / 20-30 reps
2. Back N Forth 30 sec / 1 min
3. Power (clapping) Push Ups 5 reps / 10 reps
4. Jump Rope 1 min / 1 min

Repeat all 4, no rest if possible
Beginner: 2-3x / Advanced: 2-3 x

DAY 5

OPTION 1 (QUICK WORKOUT)

Circuit 1
1. Jump Rope 1 min
2. Kettle Bell Swing 1 min / 1 min
3. Straight Bar Curls 12-15 reps (60-70%) / 12-15 reps (70-80%)
4. Hammer Curls 10-15 reps (60-70%) / 10-15 reps (70-80%)
5. **If at Gym:** Cable Curls with rope 20 reps (50%) / 20 reps (70-80%) **or if at Home**: fast blue band curls 1 min / 1 min
6. Overhead Tricep Extension, db 15-20 reps (70%) / 5 x 10 reps (90 x 80%)
7. Dips or Tricep Bench Dips till failure / till failure

Repeat all 7, no rest if possible
Beginner 1-3 x / Advanced 3-4 x

Circuit 2
1. Power Chin Ups: 30 sec / 1 min
2. Fast Hammer Curls (5-15lbs) 1 min / 1 min
3. Back N Forth 1 min / 1 min
4. Battle Rope (alternate) 1 min / 1 min

Repeat all 4, no rest if possible
Beginner: 2-3 x Advanced: 3-4 x

CARDIO
1. Boxing Level 1 (Bag) Repeat 5-10 x 2 minutes.
   Rest 1 minute or Active Rest with all 3 Exercises below In-between rounds *perform the following 3 exercises 1x:
   1. Mountain Climbers 30 sec
   2. Jumping Squats 10-20 reps
   3. High Plank 30 sec

*Once you perform all 3 exercises 1x, proceed back to boxing level 1 (bag) for a total of 5-10x.

OPTION 2 (LONGER WORKOUT)

Circuit 1
1. Jump Rope 1 min
2. Kettle Bell Swing 1 min / 1 min
3. Straight Bar Curls 12-15 reps (60-70%) / 12-15 reps (70-80%)
4. Hammer Curls 10-15 reps (60-70%) / 10-15 reps (70-80%)
5. **If at Gym:** cable curls with rope 20 reps (50%) / 5 x 5 x 5 reps (90 x 80 x 70-80%) **or if at home:** fast blue band curls 1 min / 1 min
6. Overhead Tricep Extension, db. 15-20 reps (70-80%) / drop set: 5 reps x 10 reps (90 x 80%)
7. Dips or Tricep Bench Dips till failure / till failure

Repeat all 7, no rest if possible
Beginner 1-3 x / Advanced 3-5 x

Circuit 2
1. Power Pull Ups: 30 sec / 1 min
2. Fast Hammer Curls 20 reps / (Drop Set) 5 x 5 x 5 x 5 reps (90 x 80 x 70-80%)
3. Back N' Forth 1 min / 1 min
4. Battle Rope (alternate) 1 min / 1 min

Repeat all 4, no rest if possible
Beginner: 1-2 x / Advanced: 2-3 x

CARDIO
1. Boxing Level 1 (Bag) 10 x 1-2 minute rounds
   Rest 1 min or Active Rest below between rounds by performing the following 1x only:
   1. Push Ups (power or regular) 10
   2. Mountain Climbers 30 sec

3. Jumping Squats No Weight 10- 20
4. High Plank 30 sec

Jog
Beginner 10 minutes
Advanced 20 minutes

DAY 6

OPTION 1 (QUICK WORKOUT)

CIRCUIT 1
1. Shoulder Press Straight Bar 10 reps (80%) / 10 reps (80%)
2. Shoulder Raises: Side to 45 degrees To Front Raises, dbs. 6 reps (50-60%) / 6 reps (60-80%)
3. Upright Rows 5 reps x 10 reps (80 x 70%) / drop set: 5 reps x 10 reps (90 x 80%)
4. Shrugs 15 reps (60-70%) / 6-8 reps x 10-15 reps (90% x 70%)

Repeat all 4, Beginner: 2-4 x / Advanced: 3-5 x

CIRCUIT 2
1. Push Ups elevated 5-10 reps / 10-25 reps * elevated: place knees or balls of feet on 2-12 inch elevation.
2. Sit Ups 25 / 50
3. Bicycle (abs) 30 sec / 30 sec
4. Knee Tucks (ABS) 30 sec / 1 min

Repeat all 4, Beginner: 1-3 x / Advanced: 3-5 x

CIRCUIT 3

Boxing Level 1 (bag) 3-5 X 3 minute rounds

In between rounds (3 minute rounds) perform all 3 exercises 1x:

1. Power Chin Ups 30 seconds
2. Power Pull Ups 30 seconds
3. Clapping Push Ups 30 seconds

OPTION 2 (LONGER WORKOUT)

CIRCUIT 1

1. Shoulder Press Straight Bar 10 reps (80%) / 8 reps (90%)
2. Shoulder Press dbs. (Advanced only) 5-8 reps (80%)
3. Side to Front Raises, dbs. 6 reps (50-60%) / 6 reps (60-70%)
4. Upright Rows, drop set: 5 reps x 10 reps (80 x 70%) / drop set: 5 reps x 10-12 reps (90 % x 80%)
5. Shrugs 15 reps (60-70%) / drop set: 5 reps x 15 reps (95% x 80-90%)
6. *Battle Rope, rope slam 30 sec / 1 minute

*No rope? Throw Straight Punches in air with 1-2 lbs. for same time

Repeat all 6,
Beginner: 2-3 x / Advanced: 3-5 x

CIRCUIT 2

1. Push Ups 10 reps / 25 reps
2. Sit Ups 25 / 50
3. Bicycle Abs 30 sec / 1 min
4. Knee Tucks 30 sec / 1 min

Repeat all 3,
Beginner: 2-3 x / Advanced: 4-5 x

CARDIO:

Boxing Level 1 (bag) 3-5 x 3 minute rounds

In between rounds perform:
1. Power Chin Ups 30 seconds
2. Power Pull Ups 30 seconds
3. Power Push Ups 30 seconds (knees or feet)

CIRCUIT 4

Battle Rope (alternate) or Punches in air 1 min / 2 min
Jump Rope 1 min / 3 min

Sprints:
Beginner: 10 x 25 yards
Advanced: 10 x 25 yards, 5 x 50 yards, 2 x 100 yards, jog ¼ mile

DAY 7

Rest or Cardio

Cardio:
You choose 30-90 minutes
Bike, Box, Run, Walk, etc.

DAY 8

OPTION 1 (QUICK WORKOUT)

Warm Up
1. Jumping Jacks 20
2. Bounding 30 sec
3. Star Jumps 20 / 20

Repeat all 3, 3 minutes

CIRCUIT 1:
1. Flat Chest Press, dbs. (fitness ball or bench) 5 reps (90%)
2. Incline Chest Press, dbs. (fitness ball or bench) 10 reps (70-80%)
3. Flat Flies, dbs. (fitness ball or bench) drop set: 5 reps x 5 reps (90% x 80%)
4. Push Ups or Clapping Push Ups 5 reps / 10 reps
5. Upright Rows, bar or dumbbells 6 reps (80%) / 6-8 reps (80-90%)

Repeat all 5, no rest if possible
Beginner: 1-3 x / Advanced: 2-4 x

CIRCUIT 2:
1. Jump Rope 1 min / 1 min
2. Squats Bar or Goblet Dumbbell Squat 10 reps (70% max) / 15 reps (70-80% max)
3. **If at Gym**: Leg Press 10 reps / 20 reps **or if at Home:** Jumping Squats 10 reps / 10 reps holding 20 lb. medicine ball or 20 lb. dumbbell
4. **Gym:** Back Leg Curls 10 reps (60%) / 15 reps (70%) **or if at Home:** fitness ball back leg curls 15 reps / 25 reps
5. Stand Ups 15 each leg / 25 each leg holding 10-20 lb. dumbbell horizontal under chin.

Repeat all 5, no rest if possible
Beginner: 1-3 x / Advanced: 2-4 x

OPTION 2 (LONGER WORKOUT)

Warm Up
1. Jumping Jacks 20
2. Bounding 30 sec
3. Star Jumps 20 / 20

Repeat all 3, 3 minutes

CIRCUIT 1:
1. Flat Chest Press, dbs. 8 reps (70%) / 5 reps (90%)
2. Incline Chest Press, dbs. 8 reps (60-70%) / 10 reps (70-80%)
3. Overhead pulls, dbs. 10 reps (70% max) / drop set 5 reps x 10 reps (90% x 80%)
4. Gym: Cable Flies 15 (60-70%) / 10 (80-90%) or if at Home: flat flies, dbs. 10 reps (60-70%) / 10-15 reps (80-90%)
5. Upright Rows, dbs. or bar 6 reps (80%) / 6-8 reps (80-90%)

Repeat all 5, no rest if possible
Beginner: 1-3 x / Advanced: 3-5 x

CIRCUIT 2:
1. Jump Rope 1 min / 1 min
2. Squats Bar or DB 10 reps (70% max) / 20 reps (70% max)
3. Jumping Squats 10 reps (5-10lb *mb) / 10 reps (15-25lb mb)
4. Gym: Leg Press 15 reps (60-80%) / 15-20 (80-90%) or if at Home: Walking Lunge 1 min (holding no weight) / 1 min holding 10-25 lb. dbs. in each hand.
5. Gym: Back Leg Curl 10 reps (60%) / 15 reps (70%) or if at Home: fitness ball back leg curls 15 reps/ 25 reps
6. Stand ups 10 each leg / 25 each leg holding 10-30 lb dumbbell (hold horizontal under chin).
*Mb = medicine ball

Repeat all 7, no rest if possible
Beginner: 1-3 x / Advanced: 3-4 x

CARDIO:
Jog:
Beginner 1 mile / Advanced: 2-4 miles

DAY 9

OPTION 1 (QUICK WORKOUT)

Boxing Level 1 (Bag) 3 min rounds, repeat 5x
Rest 30 sec – 1 min between rounds

No bag? Throw 2-4 punch combinations, move and repeat with or without 1-2lb. dumbbells

CIRCUIT 2:
1. Jump Rope 1 min
2. Burpees or Star Jumps 10 / 20
3. Knee Tucks 30 sec / 1 min
4. ABS: Kick Outs 30 sec / 30 sec
5. Hanging Leg raises 20 / 25-30
6. Fast High Knee Running 30 sec / 30 sec

Repeat all 6, no rest if possible
Beginner 2-3 x / Advanced 3-5 x

OPTION 2 (LONGER WORKOUT)

CIRCUIT 1
1. Boxing Level 1 (Bag) 2 minute rounds, repeat 5 – 10 x
   In between rounds perform the following 2-3x below:
   1. Push Ups or Elevated Push Ups 5-10
   2. Mountain Climbers 30 sec
   3. Squats No Weight 10

Once you perform all 3 exercises 2-3x, proceed back to boxing level 1 (bag) for a total of 5-10x.

No bag? Throw 2-4 punch combinations, move and repeat with or without 1-2lb. dumbbells.

Combination examples:

Left Jab, Straight Right, Left Hook

Left Jab, Left Jab, Straight Right

Left Jab, Straight Right, Left Hook, Straight Right

Left Jab, Right Upper Cut, Left Hook, Straight Right

2. Boxing Level 1 (foot Work) 3 min / 3 min

CIRCUIT 2:

1. Jump Rope 1 min
2. Burpees or Star Jumps 10 / 20
3. Knee Tucks 30 sec / 1 min
4. ABS: Kick Outs 30 sec / 30 sec
5. Hanging Leg raises 20 / 25-30
6. Fast High Knee Running 30 sec / 30 sec

Repeat all 6, no rest if possible

Beginner 2-3 x / Advanced 3-5 x

CARDIO:

Jog or Bike 15 - 30 minutes

DAY 10

OPTION 1 (QUICK WORKOUT)

CIRCUIT 1

1. Jump Rope 1 min
2. Straight Bar Curls 10 reps (70%) / *5 reps x 5 reps (90 x 80%)
3. Close Grip Press Triceps, bar 10 reps (60%) / 10 reps (80%)
4. Standing Curls, db (same time) 8 reps (60-70%) / 5 reps (90-95%)
5. Standing Db Curls (alternate) 5 reps (60%) / 5 reps (85-90%)

6. Tricep Rope Push Downs or Dips 10-15 reps (70%) / 15-20 reps (70%)
7. Concentration Curls 10 reps (60-70%) / 10 reps (80-90%)

*Drop Set: heavy to light weight
Repeat all 7, no rest if possible
Beginner: 1-3 x / Advanced: 3-4 x

CIRCUIT 2

1. One Arm Row 10 reps (60-80%) / 10 reps (80-90%)
2. Pull Ups till failure / till failure
3. Chin Up till failure / till failure
4. Chin Up – Hold Chin over Bar till failure / till failure
5. Shoulder Press, Bar 6 reps (70%) / 6 reps (90%)
6. Shoulder Press, dbs. 8-10 reps (50%) / 10 reps (70%)

Repeat all 6, no rest if possible
Beginner: 1-3 x / Advanced: 2-4 x

OPTION 2 (LONGER WORKOUT)

CIRCUIT 1

1. Jump Rope 1 min
2. Straight Bar Curls 10 reps / 5 reps (90%) x 5 reps (80-85%)
3. Close Grip Press Triceps 10 reps (60-70%) / 10 reps (70-80%)
4. Standing Db Curls (same time) 5 reps (80%) / 5 reps (90%)
5. Standing Db Curls (alternate) 5-10 reps (70-80%) / 5-10 reps (80-90%)
6. Gym: Tricep Rope Push Downs 10 reps (50-60%) / 10 reps (80%) or Home: Dips till failure / till failure

Repeat all 6, no rest if possible
Beginner: 1-3 x / Advanced: 4-5 x

CIRCUIT 2
1. One Arm Row 10 (60-80%) / 10 (80-90%)
2. Pull Ups till failure / till failure
3. Chin Up till failure / till failure
4. Chin Up – Hold chin over bar till failure / till failure
5. Shoulder Press Bar 10 reps (60-70%) / 10 reps (70-80%)
6. Gym: Low Row 8 reps (60%) / 8 reps (80-90%) or
   If at Home: Bent Over Raises 8-12 reps (50-70%) / 8-12 reps (70-80%)
7. Upright Rows dbs. 12 reps (60-70%) / drop set: 5 reps x 5 reps x 5 reps (90 x 80-90 x 70-80%)
8. Shrugs 12-15 reps (60-70%) / 12-15 reps (70-80%)

Repeat all 8, no rest if possible
Beginner: 1-2 x / Advanced: 3-4 x

Cardio:

Beginner
Jog 1 mile
Sprints:
4 x 25 yards (rest with a walk back)
3 x 50 yards (rest with a walk back)

Can't run outside? Run on treadmill 15 minutes with sprint 30 sec every other minute.

Advanced:
Jog 1 mile
Sprints:
5 x 25 yards (rest with trot back)
5 x 50 yards (rest with trot back)
5 x 100 yards (rest with trot back)

Can't run outside? Run on treadmill 20 minutes with sprint 1 min every other minute.

DAY 11

OPTION 1 (QUICK WORKOUT)

CIRCUIT 1:
1. Flat Press Bench 5 reps (80%) / 5 reps (90%)
2. Incline Press Bench 5 reps (80-90%) / 5 reps (90%)
3. **If at Home:** Flat Flies, dbs. or **if at Gym:** Cable Flies 10 reps (70%) / drop set: 5 rep x 10 reps (95% x 70%)
4. Incline Flies, Dbs. 15 reps / 15 reps
5. Air Squats 20 reps / 20 reps

Repeat all 5, no rest if possible
Beginner: 1-2 x / Advanced: 2-4 x

CIRCUIT 2
1. Squats, dumbbell or Bar 10 reps (50%) / 10 reps (50%)
2. Dips till failure / till failure

CIRCUIT 3
1. Bar Squats or Goblet Db, drop set: 5 reps x 5 reps (80% x 70%) / drop set: 5 reps x 5-8 reps (90% x 80%)
2. **If at Gym:** leg press 10-15 reps (70%) / 15-20 reps (80%) **or if at Home** alternate lunges 10 reps each leg holding a db in each hand (i.e. 10-15lbs) / 10 reps each leg holding a db in each hand (i.e 15-30lbs.)
3. **If at Gym:** back leg curl 8 reps (50%) / 12 reps (70%) **or if at home,** back leg curl w fitness ball 15 reps / 20 reps
4. Hanging leg raises 20 reps / 25 reps
5. Plank 1 min / 1 min
6. 45 degree Crunches 30 sec / 30 sec
7. Bicycle 30 sec / 30 sec

8. Push Ups 10 reps / 20 reps

Repeat all 8, no rest if possible
Beginner: 1-3 x / Advanced: 2-4 x

CIRCUIT 4
1. Punches: left, Right (punch over eye level – Fast) 1 min / 1 min
2. Mountain climbers 1 min / 2 min
3. Punches: hooks to head - Fast 1 min / 1 min
4. Jump Rope or Jumping Jacks 1 min / 1 min
5. Punches: Upper Cuts to Head - Fast 1 min / 1 min

Repeat all 5, no rest if possible
Beginner: 1-2 x /Advanced: 2 x

OPTION 2 (LONGER WORKOUT)

CIRCUIT 1:
1. Flat Press Bench or Fitness Ball 5 reps (80%) / 5 reps (90%)
2. Incline Press Bench or Ball 5 reps (80-90%) / 5 reps (90%)
3. Incline Flies 15 reps / 15 reps
4. **If at Home:** flat flies, dbs. or **if at Gym:** cable flies drop set *5 reps x 10 reps (80-90% x 70-80%) / drop set: 10 reps x 10 reps (90% x 80%)

Repeat all 4, no rest if possible
Beginner: 1-3 x / Advanced: 3-4 x

CIRCUIT 2
1. Squats bar or Goblet db 10 reps (50%) / 10 reps (50%)
2. Dips till failure / till failure

CIRCUIT 3
1. Squat Bar or Goblet 10 reps (50%) / 10 reps (50 %)

2. Squats Bar or Goblet, drop set: 5 reps x 5 reps (80% x 70%) / 5 reps x 5-8 reps (90% x 80%)
3. **If at Home:** Good Mornings 10 reps / 10 reps **or if at the Gym**: Back Leg Curls 8 reps (50-60 %) / 10-15 reps (70-80%)
4. Jumping Squats 10 / 20 reps holding medicine ball (10-20lb.) at chest under chin entire time.
5. Hanging leg raises or Leg Raises 20 reps / 25 reps
6. Plank 1 min / 1 min
7. Sit Ups 25 / 50
8. Kick Outs 30 sec / 30 sec
9. Push Ups 10 reps / 25 reps

Repeat all 9, no rest if possible
Beginner: 2-3 x / Advanced: 3-5 x

CIRCUIT 4
1. Punches: left, Right (punch over eye level – Fast) 1 min / 1 min
2. Mountain climbers 1 min / 1 min
3. Punches: hooks to head - Fast 1 min / 1min
4. Jumping Jacks 1 min / 1min
5. Punches: Upper Cuts to Head - Fast 1 min / 1 min
6. Run High Knee 1 min / 1 min
7. 3 straights, 2 hooks, 1 upper cuts 1 min / 1 min

Repeat all 7, no rest if possible
Beginner: 1-2 x / Advanced: 2 x

CARDIO
1. Burpees or Star Jumps 10 reps / 30 reps
2. Power Push Ups 5-10 / 20-50
3. Jump Rope 1 min / 1 min
4. Mountain Climbers 1 min / 1 min

Repeat all 4, no rest if possible
Beginner 1-2 x / Advanced 2-3 x

DAY 12

OPTION 1 (QUICK WORKOUT)

Circuit 1
1. Jump Rope 1 min
2. Kettle Bell Swing 1 min / 1 min
3. Straight Bar Curls 12-15 reps (60%) / drop set: 5 reps x 10 reps (90% x 80%)
4. Hammer Curls 10-15 reps (70%) / drop set: 5 reps x 10-15 reps (90% 70%%)
5. Overhead Tricep Extension, db 15-20 reps (70%) / drop set: 5 reps x 10-15 reps (90 x 80-90%)
6. Dips or tricep bench dips till failure / till failure

Repeat all 6, no rest if possible
Beginner 2-3 x, Advanced 2-5 x

Circuit 2
1. Power Chin Ups: 30 sec / 30 sec 1 min
2. Fast Curls w band (blue) or dumbbells (10-15lbs): 1 min / 1 min

Repeat Both, no rest if possible
Beginner: 2-3 x Advanced: 3-4 x

CARDIO
1. Boxing Level 1 (Bag) 5 x 2-3 minutes
   Active Rest between rounds by performing the following 1 x:
2. Push Ups or Elevated Push Ups 10
3. Mountain Climbers 30 sec
4. Jumping Squats reps 20

OPTION 2 (LONGER WORKOUT)

CIRCUIT 1
1. Jump Rope 1 min
2. Kettle Bell Swing 1 min / 1 min
3. Straight Bar Curls 12-15 reps (60%) /drop set: 5 reps x 10 - 12reps (90 x 80%)
4. Hammer Curls 10-15 reps (70%) / 10-15 reps (70-80%)
5. Overhead Tricep Extension, db. 15-20 reps (70%) / drop set: 5 reps x 10-15 reps (90 x 80-90%)
6. Tricep Push Ups 5-10 / 10-20

Repeat all 6, no rest if possible
Beginner 3 x / Advanced 3-6 x

CIRCUIT 2
1. Jumping Pull Ups: 30 sec / 1 min
2. Fast Curls w band (blue): 1 min / 1 min

Repeat Both, no rest if possible
Beginner: 2-3 x / Advanced: 3-4 x

CARDIO
1. Boxing Level 1 (Bag) 5-10 x 2 minute rounds
   Active Rest between rounds by performing the following:
   1. Push Ups 10 reps
   2. Mountain Climbers 30 sec
   3. Jumping Squats holding 20 reps

Jog
Beginner 10-20 minutes
Advanced 20 – 30 minutes

DAY 13

OPTION 1 (QUICK WORKOUT)

CIRCUIT 1
1. Shoulder Press Straight Bar 10 reps (60-70%) / 5 reps (70-80%)
2. Shoulder Press (dbs.) advanced only 5 reps (70-80%)
3. Shoulder Raises: Side to 45 degrees to Front Raises, dbs. 5 reps (60%) / 6-8 reps (70-80%)
4. Upright Rows drop set: 5 reps x 5 reps (80 x 70-80%) / drop set: 5 reps x 5 reps x 5-10 reps (90% x 80-90 % x 70-80%)
5. Shrugs 15 reps (60-70%) /10 reps x 10 reps (80-90% x 70-80%)
6. Battle Rope (alternate) 30 sec / 1 min
7. Battle Rope (slams) 20 reps / 30 reps
* no rope? Perform Straight overhead punches w 1-2lbs for 1 minute
Repeat all 7, Beginner: 2-4 x / Advanced: 3-5 x

CIRCUIT 2
1. Straight Bar Curls 12 reps (70%) / 6 reps x 6 reps (90% x 80-90%)
2. Concentration Curls 10 reps (70%) / 10 reps (90%) Heavy: assist with other hand if failing
3. Push Ups 10 reps / 25 reps
4. Leg Raises or Hanging Leg Raises 25 / 50
5. 45 degree Crunches 30 sec / 30 sec
6. Hops 30 sec / 1 min

Repeat all 6, Beginner: 2-4 x / Advanced: 3-4 x
Boxing Level 1 (bag) 2-3 x 3 minute rounds

Active Rest In-between 3 minute rounds, perform all 3 exercises 1x:
1. Jumping Chin Ups 30 seconds
2. Jumping Pull Ups 30 seconds
3. Clapping Push Ups 30 seconds

OPTION 2 (LONGER WORKOUT)

CIRCUIT 1

1. Shoulder Press Straight Bar 10 reps (60-70%) / 10 reps (70-80%)
2. Side to 45 degrees to Front Raises, dbs. 5 reps (60%) / 6-8 (70-80%)
3. Upright Rows 5 reps x 5 reps (80 x 70-80%) / 5 reps x 5 reps x 5 reps (90 x 80-90 x 70-80%)
4. Shrugs 15 reps (60-70%) / 10 reps x 10-15 reps (80-90% x 70-80%)
5. Battle Rope alternate 30 sec /1 minute or if no rope, Straight overhead punches w 1-2lbs for 1 minute
6. Battle Rope (slams) 20 reps / 30 reps

Repeat all 6,
Beginner: 2-3 x / Advanced: 2-4 x

CIRCUIT 2:

1. Straight Bar Curls12 reps / 6 reps x 6 reps Heavy to light, drop set
2. Concentration Curls10 reps / 10 reps Heavy: assist with other hand if failing
3. Push Ups 10 reps / 25 reps
4. Bent Over Raises 10 reps (50-60%) / 10-15 reps (70-80%)
5. **If at Gym:** Close Grip Pull Down 10 reps (70%) / 8 reps (80-90%)
6. Hanging Leg raises (abs) 20-30 / 30-50
7. **If at Gym:** low rows 10 reps (80%) / 5-8 reps (90%)

Repeat all 7,
Beginner: 2-3 x / Advanced: 3-4 x

CIRCUIT 3:

Boxing Level 1 (bag) 3 minute rounds, repeat 3x

Active Rest In-between rounds perform all 3 exercises, 1x:
1. Power Chin Ups 30 seconds
2. Power Pull Ups 30 seconds
3. Clapping Push Ups 30 seconds

CIRCUIT 4
1. Battle Rope (rope slam) 30 / 50
2. Jump Rope: 1 min / 2 min
3. Knee Tucks 30 sec / 1 min

Repeat All 3, no rest if possible
Beginner: 1x / Advanced: 1-2x

Sprints:
Beginner: 10 x 25 yards, 2 x 100 yards
Advanced: 10 x 25 yards, 5 x 50 yards, 2 x 100 yards, jog 1/2 mile

DAY 14

Rest or Cardio

Cardio:
You choose 30-90 minutes
Bike, Box, Run, Walk, etc…

DAY 15

OPTION 1 (QUICK WORKOUT)
Warm Up
1. Jumping Jacks 30
2. Push Ups or Power Push Ups 5-10
3. Sit Ups 20
4. Stand ups 5 each leg

Repeat all 4, 5 minutes (no rest)

CIRCUIT 1:
1. Flat Chest Press, dbs. with fitness ball or bar with bench 6-8 reps (80-90%)/ 4-6 reps (90-95%)
2. Leg Lifts 25 reps / 50 reps

Repeat both, no rest if possible
Beginner: 3 x / Advanced: 4 x

CIRCUIT 2:
1. Incline Chest Press, dbs. with fitness ball or bar with bench 8-10 reps (70-80%) / 8-10 reps (80-90%)
2. Plank 1-2 min / 2 min

Repeat both, no rest if possible
Beginner: 2-3 x / Advanced: 4 x

CIRCUIT 3:
1. **If at Home: Flat** Flies dbs. (home) **or if at gym:** Cable Flies drop set: 8 reps x 12 or great reps till burn (90% x 70%)
2. Overhead Pulls 10 reps (80% max) / 10-15 reps (80-90% max)
3. Mountain Climbers 1 min / 2 min

Repeat all 3, no rest if possible
Beginner: 1 x / Advanced: 2-3 x

CIRCUIT 4:
1. Jump Rope 1 min / 1 min
2. Squats with Bar or Goblet Db. 20 reps (70% max) / 20 reps (70-80% max)
3. **Gym:** Leg Press 10 reps (80-90%) / drop set: 10 reps x 10 reps (90% x 80%) or **if at home:** Jumping Squats 10 reps with 10lb medicine ball / 15-25 reps with 20 lb. medicine ball

4. **Home:** Good Mornings or **if at Gym:** Back Leg Curl 10 reps (80%) / drop set: 10 reps x 10 reps (90% x 80%)
5. Run High Knee 1 min / 2 min

Repeat all 5, no rest if possible
Beginner: 1-2 x / Advanced: 3-4 x

OPTION 2 (LONGER WORKOUT)
Warm Up
1. Jumping Jacks 30
2. Push Ups or Power Push Ups 5-10
3. Sit Ups 20
4. Stand Ups 5 each leg

Repeat all 4, 5-10 minutes (no rest)

CIRCUIT 1
1. Flat Chest Press, dbs with fitness ball or bar with bench 6-8 reps (80-90%)/ 4-6 reps (90-95%)
2. Leg Lifts 25 reps / 50 reps

Repeat both, no rest if possible
Beginner: 3 x / Advanced: 4 x

CIRCUIT 2:
1. Incline Chest Press, dbs with fitness ball or bar with bench 8-10 reps (70-80%) / 8-10 reps (80-90%)
2. Plank 1-2 min / 2 min

Repeat both, no rest if possible
Beginner: 3 x / Advanced: 4 x

CIRCUIT 3:
1. **If at Home:** Flat Flies Dbs 10 reps (80%) / 10 reps (90%) **or if at gym:** Cable Flies, drop set: 8 reps x 12 reps or till burn (90% x 70%)
2. Overhead Pulls 10 reps (80%) / 10-15 reps (80-90%)

Repeat both, no rest if possible
Beginner: 1 x / Advanced: 2-3 x

CIRCUIT 4:
1. Jump Rope or Jumping Jacks 1 min / 1 min
2. Squats (Bar or Dumbbell) 5 reps (80%) / 8 reps (80-90%)
3. Squats (Bar or Dumbbell) 10-15 reps (70%) / 10-15 reps (70-80%)
4. Jumping Squats 10 with 10lb medicine ball / 10-20 reps holding a 20 lb. medicine ball
5. Stretch legs 2 min

Repeat all 5, no rest if possible
Beginner: 1-3 x / Advanced: 4-5 x

CIRCUIT 5:
1. **If at Home:** Good Mornings **or if at the Gym:** Back Leg Curl 10 reps (80%) / drop set: 5 reps x 10 reps (90% x 80%)
2. **If at Home:** Alternate Lunges 10 reps each side (holding 10-15 lbs. in each hand) / 12 reps each side (holding 20-30lbs in each hand) **or if at the Gym:** Leg Press 10 reps (80%) / 8 reps x 8-12 reps (90% x 80%)

Repeat both, no rest if possible
Beginner: 1-3 x / Advanced: 4-5 x

CARDIO:
Jog:
Beginner 1 mile

Advanced: 2-4 miles

DAY 16

OPTION 1 (QUICK WORKOUT)
Boxing Level 1 (Bag) 3 min rounds, repeat 5x
Rest 30 sec – 1 min between rounds
No bag? Throw 2-4 punch combinations, move and repeat with or without 1-2lb. dumbbells

Circuit 2:
1. Jump Rope 1 min
2. Plank 1 min
3. Back N Forth 1 min
4. Knee Tucks 30 sec
5. Pull Ups till failure / till failure
6. Power Chin Ups 30 sec

Repeat all 6, no rest if possible
Beginner 2-4x / Advanced 4-5 x

CARDIO
Sprints
Beginner: 10 x 25 yards

Advanced: 10 x 25 yards, 10 x 50 yards

OPTION 2 (LONGER WORKOUT)

CIRCUIT 1
1. Boxing Level 1 (Bag) 5 x 2 min rounds

In between rounds perform the following 3 exercises, 1x:
1. Knee Tucks 25
2. Mountain Climbers 1 min
3. Air Squats (No Weight) 25

No bag? Throw 2-4 punch combinations, move and repeat with or without 1-2lb. dumbbells.
Combination examples:

- Left Jab, Straight Right, Left Hook
- Left Jab, Left Jab, Straight Right
- Left Jab, Straight Right, Left Hook, Straight Right
- Left Jab, Right Upper Cut, Left Hook, Straight Right

CIRCUIT 2:
Boxing Level 1 (foot Work) 3 min / 3 min

CIRCUIT 3:
1. Jump Rope 1 min
2. High Knee Running 1 min / 1 min
3. Jumping Squats 10 reps / 10 reps
4. Knee Tucks 30 sec / 1 min
5. Kick Outs 30 sec / 30 sec
5. Pull Ups till failure / till failure
6. Power Chin Ups 30 sec / 30 sec

Repeat all 6, no rest if possible
Beginner 2-4 x / Advanced 3-6 x

CARDIO:
Beginner
Sprints: 10 x 25 yards
Jog or Bike 15 min

Advanced:
Sprints: 10 x 25 yards, 10 x 50 yards
Jog or Bike 30 minutes

DAY 17

OPTION 1 (QUICK WORKOUT)

CIRCUIT 1
1. Jump Rope 1 min
2. Straight Bar Curls 6 reps (80%) / drops set: 5 reps x 5 reps (90% x 80%)
3. Close Grip Tricep press 6 reps (80%) / 6 reps (90%)

4. Standing Db Curls (same time) 8 reps (60-70%) / 5 reps (90-95%)
5. Standing Db Curls (alternate) 5 reps (60%) / 5 reps (85-90%)
6. **If at Gym:** Tricep Rope Push Downs 10-15 reps (80-90%) / 15-20 (80-90%) **or if at Home:** Dips or Tricep Bench Dips till failure / till failure
7. Concentration Curls 10 reps (80%) / drop set: 5 reps x 10 reps (90% x 80%)

Repeat all 7, no rest if possible
Beginner: 2-3 x / Advanced: 4-5 x

CIRCUIT 2
1. One Arm Row 10 reps (60-80%) / 6 reps (80-90%)
2. Shoulder Press dbs. 6 reps (80%) / 4-6 reps (90%)
3. **Gym:** Low Rows 8 reps (70-80%) / 6-8 reps (80-90**%) or if at Home:** Bent Over Raises 10 reps (60%) / 10 reps (80%)

Repeat all 3, no rest if possible
Beginner: 2-4 x, Advanced: 4-6 x

CIRCUIT 3
1. **Gym:** Close Grip Pulls 6 reps (80%) / 6-8 reps (80-90%) or **if at Home:** chin ups till failure / till failure
2. **Gym:** Wide Grip Pulls 6 reps (80%) / 6-8 reps (80-90%)
3. Chin Ups: till failure / till failure
4. 1 Chin Up with hold till failure / till failure
5. Side Raises to 45 degrees to front raises (dbs.) 8 reps (70%) / 8 reps (80-90%)
6. Upright Rows 6 reps (80%) / 6-8 reps (80-90%)

Repeat all 6, no rest if possible
Beginner: 2-3 x / Advanced: 3-4 x

OPTION 2 (LONGER WORKOUT)

CIRCUIT 1
1. Jump Rope 1 min

2. Straight Bar Curls 6 reps (80%) / drop set: 5 reps x 5 reps (90 x 80%)
3. Close Grip Tricep Press 6 reps (80%) / 6 reps (90%)
4. Standing Db Curls (same time) 8 reps (70-80%) / 5 reps (90-95%)
5. Standing Db Curls (alternate) 5 reps (70%) / 5 reps (85-90%)
6. **Gym:** Tricep Rope Push Downs 10-15 reps / 15-20 reps
   or if at Home: Dips till failure / till failure
7. Concentration Curls 10 reps (80%) / drop set: 5 reps x 10 reps (95% x 80%)

Repeat all 7, no rest if possible
Beginner: 1-3 x / Advanced: 3-5 x

CIRCUIT 2
1. One Arm Row 10 reps (60-80%) / 6 reps (90%)
2. Shoulder Press dbs. 6-8 reps (80%) / 6-8 reps (90%)
3. Shoulder Press bar 5-8 reps (70%) / 5-8 reps (70-80%)
4. **Gym:** Low Rows 8-12 reps (70-80%) / 8-12 reps (80%) **or if at Home:** bent over raises 10 reps (60%) / 10 reps (80%)

Repeat all 4, no rest if possible
Beginner: 2-4 x / Advanced: 4-6 x

CIRCUIT 3
1. **Gym:** Close Grip Pulls (gym) 6 reps (80%) / 6-8 reps (80-90%) **or if at Home**: chin ups till failure / till failure
2. **Gym**: Wide Grip Pulls 6 reps (80%) / 6-8reps (80-90%) **or if at home:** pull ups till failure
3. Chin Ups: till failure / till failure * if you performed chin ups at home above, perform 1 chin up and hold chin over bar as long as you can.
4. 1 Chin Up with hold till failure / till failure
5. Side Raises to 45 degrees to front raises (dbs.) 8 reps (70%) / 8 reps (80-90%)
6. Upright Rows, bar 10 reps (60%) / 6-8 reps (80%)
7. Shrugs, bar 12 reps (80%) / drop set: 6 reps x 8-10 reps (90% x 70%)

Repeat all 6, no rest if possible
Beginner: 1-3 x / Advanced: 3-4 x

CARDIO:
Beginner:
Jog 1 mile
Sprints:
1. 10 x 25 yards (rest with a walk back)
2. 6 x 50 yards (rest with a walk back)

Can't run outside? Run on treadmill 15 minutes with sprint 30 sec every other minute.

Advanced:
Jog 1 mile
Sprints:
5. x 25 yards (rest with trot back)
5. x 50 yards (rest with trot back)
5. x 100 yards (rest with trot back)

Can't run outside? Run on treadmill 20 minutes with sprint 1 min every other minute.

DAY 18

OPTION 1 (QUICK WORKOUT)

CIRCUIT 1:
1. Flat Press Bench or Fitness Ball 5 reps (80%) / 5 reps (90%)
2. Incline Press Bench or Ball 5 reps (80-90%) / 5 reps (90%)
3. **If at Home:** Flat Flies, Dbs. **or if at Gym:** Cable Flies 10 reps (70%) / drop set: 5 reps x 10 reps (95% x 70%)
4. Close Grip Tricep Press 10-15 reps (60-70%) / 10 reps (80%)
5. Dips till failure / till failure
6. Overhead Pull Overs 10 reps (80%) / drop set: 5 reps (90%) x 10 reps (80-90%)

Repeat all 6, no rest if possible

Beginner: 2-3 x / Advanced: 3-4 x

CIRCUIT 2
1. Squats bar or Goblet dumbbell 5 reps (80%) / 5 reps (80-90%)
2. Squats Bar or Goblet 5 reps (70%) / 10 reps (70-80%)
3. **Gym:** Leg Press 10 reps (80-90%) / 8 x 10 (80-90 x 70-80%) or **Home:** stand ups 25 each leg / 20 each leg holding 10-20 lbs
4. **Gym:** back leg curls 10 (80-90%) / 10 (80-90%) or **Home:** good mornings 10 / 10 and fitness ball back leg curls 10 / 15
5. Hanging leg raises 20 / 25
6. Push Ups 10 / 20

Repeat all 6, no rest if possible
Beginner: 1-3 x, Advanced: 3-5 x

CIRCUIT 3
1. Punches: left, Right over eye level - Fast 1 min / 1 min
2. Mountain climbers 1 min / 1 min
3. Punches: hooks to head - Fast 1 min / 1min
4. Jumping Jacks 1 min / 1min
5. Punches: Upper Cuts to Head - Fast 1 min / 1 min

Repeat all 5, no rest if possible
Beginner: 1-2 x, Advanced: 2 x

OPTION 2 (LONGER WORKOUT)

CIRCUIT 1:
1. Flat Press Bench or Fitness Ball 5 reps (80%) / 5 reps (90%)
2. Incline Press Bench or Ball 5 reps (80-90%) / 5 reps (90%)
3. Incline Flies 15 reps / 15 reps
4. **Home:** Flat Bench Flies or **Gym:** Cables *5 x 10 (70-80%) / 5 x 10 (90 x 80%) * drop sets. Start with heaviest weight and drop down every 5 reps.
5. Overhead Pull Overs 10 reps (80%) / drop set: 5 reps (90%) x 10 reps (80-90%)

You should be struggling with each exercise of only 5 reps.

Repeat all 5, no rest if possible
Beginner: 2-3 x / Advanced: 3-4 x

CIRCUIT 2
1. Squats bar or Goblet dumbbell 5 reps (80%) / 5 reps (80-90%)
2. Squats Bar or Goblet 5 reps (70%) / 10 reps (70%)
3. **Gym:** Leg Press 10 (70%) / 20 (80-90%) or **Home:** stand ups 25 each leg / 20 each leg holding 10-20 lbs.
4. **Gym:** Back Leg Curls 10 reps (80 %) / 10 reps (80-90%) or **Home:** Good Mornings 10 / 10 and fitness ball back leg curls 10 / 15
5. Hanging leg raises 20 / 25
6. Bench Step Ups 10 each leg holding 10-15lb dbs / 10 each leg holding 15-20 lb dbs
7. Plank 1 min / 1 min
8. Close Grip Press Tricep press 10-15 reps (60-70%) / 10 reps (80%)
9. Dips till Failure / Till Failure

Repeat all 9, no rest if possible
Beginner: 2-3 x / Advanced: 3-4 x

CIRCUIT 3
1. Punches: left, Right over eye level - Fast 1 min / 1 min
2. Mountain climbers 1 min / 1 min
3. Punches: hooks to head - Fast 1 min / 1min
4. Jumping Jacks 1 min / 1min
5. Punches: Upper Cuts to Head - Fast 1 min / 1 min
6. Run High Knee 1 min / 1 min
7. 3 straights, 2 hooks, 2 upper cuts 1 min / 1 min

Repeat all 7, no rest if possible
Beginner: 1-2 x / Advanced: 2 x

CARDIO
1. Burpees or Star Jumps 10-15 / 30
2. Power Push Ups 5 / 20
3. Jump Rope 1 min / 1 min

4. Mountain Climbers 1 min / 1 min
5. Jumping Squats 5 / 10

Repeat all 5, no rest if possible
Beginner 1-3 x / Advanced 2-3 x

DAY 19

OPTION 1 (QUICK WORKOUT)

Circuit 1
1. Jump Rope 1 min
2. Kettle Bell Swing 1 min / 1 min
3. Sit Ups 25 / 50
4. Hanging Leg Raises or Leg Raises 20 / 30

Repeat all 4, no rest if possible
Beginner 2-3 x / Advanced 4-6 x

Circuit 2
1. **Gym:** Low Row 10-15 reps (70%) / 8-12 reps (70-90%)
2. **Gym: Gravitron** Pull Ups, 15-20 reps (70-80%) / 15-20 (70-80%) **Home:** Pull Ups till failure / till failure
3. Dips or Tricep Bench till failure / till failure

Repeat all 3, no rest if possible
Beginner 2-3 x / Advanced 3-5 x

Circuit 3
1. Jumping Pull Ups: 30 sec / 1 min
2. Mountain Climbers 30 sec / 30 sec

Repeat both, no rest if possible
Beginner: 2-3 x Advanced: 3-4 x

CARDIO
1. Boxing Level 1 (Bag) 10 x 2 minute rounds
   Active Rest between rounds by performing the following:

1. Push Ups or Elevated Push Ups 5-10
2. Mountain Climbers 30 sec
3. Jumping Squats No Weight 20

OPTION 2 (LONGER WORKOUT)

Circuit 1
1. Jump Rope 1 min
2. Kettle Bell Swing 1 min / 1 min
3. One Arm Rows 8 reps (70-90%) / 8 reps (80-90%)

Repeat all 3, no rest if possible
Beginner 2-3 x / Advanced 3-6 x

Circuit 2
1. **Gym**: Low Row 10-15 (70%) / 8-12 (70-90%)
2. **Gym:** gravitron Pull Ups, 15-20 (70-80%) / 15-20 (70-80%)
   or **Home:** Pull Ups till failure / till failure
3. Bent Over Raises 12 (50-60%) / 5 x 10 (90 x 60%)
4. **Gym:** Wide Grip Pull Down 6 reps (90%) / 6 reps (90%)
   or **Home** Power Pull Ups 30 sec / 1 min
5. Dips or Tricep Bench till failure / till failure

Repeat all 5, no rest if possible
Beginner 2-3 x / Advanced 4-6 x

Circuit 3
3. Jumping Pull Ups: 30 sec / 1 min
4. Close Grip Pull Down 10 (80-90%) / 5 x 8 (90 x 80-90%)
5. Crunches 25 - 50
6. Wide Grip Pull Downs 10 (70-90%) / 5 x 8 (90 x 80-90%)

Repeat Both, no rest if possible
Beginner: 2-3 x / Advanced: 3-4 x

CARDIO
1. Boxing Level 1 (Bag) 3-5 x 2-3 minute rounds

Active Rest between rounds by performing the following:

1. Push Ups 10
2. Mountain Climbers 30 sec
3. Jumping Squats No Weight 25 reps

Jog
Beginner 5-10 minutes

Advanced 20 – 30 minutes

DAY 20

OPTION 1 (QUICK WORKOUT)

Circuit 1
1. Shoulder Press Straight Bar 10 reps (60-70%) / 10 reps (70-80%)
2. Side to Front Raises, dbs. 5 reps (60%) / 5 reps (70-80%)
3. Upright Rows 5 reps x 5 reps (80 x 70-80%) / 5 reps x 5 reps x 5 reps (90 x 80-90 x 70-80%)
4. Shrugs 15 reps (60-70%) / 10 reps x 10 reps (80-90% x 70-80%)

Repeat all 4,
Beginner: 2-4 x / Advanced: 3-6 x

Circuit 2
1. Straight Bar Curls 12 reps (70%) / 6 reps x 6 reps (90% x 80-90%)
2. Concentration Curls 10 reps / 10 reps (90%) Heavy: assist with other hand if failing
3. Close Grip Press 10 reps (70%) / 6-8 reps (80%)
4. Push Ups 10 reps / 25 reps

Repeat all 3, Beginner: 2-4 x / Advanced: 3-5 x

Option:
Boxing Level 1 (bag) 3 x 3 minute rounds
In between rounds (3 minutes) perform:
1. Power Chin Ups 30 seconds
2. Power Pull Ups 30 seconds
3. Clapping Push Ups 30 seconds

Repeat all 3 exercises, Beginner: 1x / Advanced: 2x

OPTION 2 (LONGER WORKOUT)

CIRCUIT 1
1. Shoulder Press straight Bar 10 reps (60-70%) / 10 reps (70-80%)
2. Shoulder Raises Side To 45 degrees to Front Raises, dbs 5 reps (60%) / 5 reps (70-80%)
3. Upright Rows 5 reps x 5 reps (80% x 70-80%) / 5 reps x 5 reps x 5 reps (90% x 80-90 % x 70-80%)
4. Shrugs 15 (60-70%) / 10 reps x 10 reps (80-90% x 70-80%)
5. Battle Rope slam 30 reps / 50 reps

Repeat all 5, Beginner: 2-4 x / Advanced: 3-5 x

CIRCUIT 2
1. Straight Bar Curls 12 reps / 6 reps x 6 reps Heavy to light, drop set
2. Concentration Curls 10 reps / 10 reps Heavy: assist with other hand if failing
3. Close Grip Press 10 reps (80%) / 6 reps (80-90%)
4. Bent Over Raises 10 reps (60-80%) / 10-12 reps (80-90%)

Repeat all 4, Beginner: 3-4 x / Advanced: 4-6 x

CARDIO:
Boxing Level 1 (bag) 3 x 3 minutes
In between rounds (3 minutes) perform:
1. Jumping Chin Ups 30 seconds
2. Jumping Pull Ups 30 seconds
3. Clapping Push Ups 30 seconds
4. Hammer Curls 20 reps (60%) / 30 reps (60-70%)

Repeat all 4 exercises, Beginner: 1 x / Advanced: 1 x

Battle Rope (alternate)
Beginner: 1 minute

Advanced: 2 minutes (alternate min 1, rope slam for min 2)
No rope? Throw straight punches with 1-2 lb. dumbbells

Jump Rope:
Beginner and advanced: 3 minutes

Sprints:
Beginner: 10 x 25 yards, 2 x 100 yards

Advanced: 10 x 25 yards, 5 x 50 yards, 2 x 100 yards, jog 1/2 mile

DAY 21

Rest or Cardio
Cardio:
You choose 30-90 minutes

Bike, Box, Run, Walk, etc...
You Made It!

Hopefully you were able to perform all 21 days. Preferably the longer workouts.

What to do next?

2 Options:
Option 1: Go back and repeat phase 1 or Perform the advanced level for phase 2.
Option 2: Get a personal program or coaching with me to create a custom program that's tailored just for you. A program that fits into your lifestyle, goals, etc..

Simply, email me at bsstudio@comcast.net and get a Free Consultation. Just use this subject line: "Double My Fitness." Then tell me your short-term and long-term goals.

3 BONUS TRAVELING WORKOUTS

Workout #1:
1. Jog 1 mile
2. Squat   25-50
3. Push Ups   10-25
4. Run High Knee   1 min – 2 min
5. Sit Ups   25 – 50
6. Leg Lifts   20-50

Repeat all above 5 x

WORKOUT #2
1. Jumping Jacks w fist   50 – 100
2. Squat   25 – 50
3. Jumping Squat   10 – 25
4. Back N Forth   1 min – 2 min
5. Push Ups   10 – 25
6. Mountain Climbers   1 – 2 min
7. Bicycle (abs)   30 sec – 1 min
8. Plank   1 min – 2 min
9. Wall Sit   Till Failure

Repeat all above 4 – 5 x

WORKOUT #3

Circuit 1
1. Squat, bar or dumbbell   8 reps
2. Jumping Squat   10-25
3. Sit ups   25-50

Repeat all 4x, no rest

Circuit 2
1. Flat press, dbs or bar   10 reps
2. Standing Curls, bar   12 reps
3. Pull Ups   till failure

Repeat all 4-5x, no rest

Circuit 3
1. Push Ups   10-50
2. Jumping Jacks or Rope   1 min

Repeat 4-5x, no rest

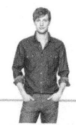

GUY #2 (LADY KILLER)
GYM Required

WARNING: These workouts are 60-90 minutes each! However it's only 21 days. You can do this. Pull your man card out.

Are you ready to pack on muscle and get laid? This won't make you look like a meat head in 21 Days but will definitely help you go from skinny to fit or obese to pudgy. You may even become a closet poser in a little thong checking out your new body.

Your results will be in line with the efforts you put into each workout. You're wasting your time if you just walk around the gym looking at yourself.

You need to train with intensity and push each rep to the max. The last 2-3 reps should be a struggle (good form obviously). If the last 2-3 reps aren't challenging, go up in weight and train harder.

If any workout is too long or your short on time. Perform at least 2 sets of each circuit. **Don't skip a workout if possible.** However, you must lift heavy. A spotter may be needed with certain lifts.

PHASE 2

WEEK 1

DAY 1

CIRCUIT 1
1. *Flat Bench Press, bar 8 reps (70%) / 8 reps (70%)
2. Crunches 25 reps / 50 reps

Repeat both, no rest if possible
Beginner 1 x / Advanced 1 x
*Use dumbbells if you have a shoulder problem

CIRCUIT 2
1. Flat Bench Press 5 reps (80%) / 5-6 reps (90%)
2. Leg Lifts 25 / 50

Repeat both, no rest if possible
Beginner 1 x, Advanced 3 x

CIRCUIT 3
1. Incline press, dbs. 8 reps (60%) / 8-10 reps (80%)
2. Close Grip Press: bar 10 reps (60%) / 10-12 reps (60-70%)
3. Push down tricep (rope or straight bar) 20 reps (60%) / 8 reps x
   20-25 reps (80-90% x 60-70%)

Repeat all 3, no rest if possible
Beginner 1 x / Advanced 3 x

CIRCUIT 4
1. Squat (free bar or smith machine) 10 reps (50%) / 10 reps (70%)
2. Back Leg Curls 10 reps (70%) / 12 reps (70%)
3. Leg extension 25 reps / 25 reps

Repeat all 3, no rest if possible
Beginner 2 x / Advanced 2 x

CIRCUIT 5 (advanced only)
1. Squat (free bar or smith machine) 8 reps (80-90%)
2. Overhead Pulls (chest) 8-10 reps (90%)
3. Leg Press 20-30 reps (70-80%)

Repeat all 3, rest 2 min between repeating circuit, stretch after leg press.

Advanced Only 3 - 4 x

CARDIO
Bike, Step Mill or Stair Master 15 minutes

DAY 2

CIRCUIT 1
1. Straight Bar Curls 8 reps (80%) / 8 reps (80%)
2. Standing Front Shoulder Press Bar 10 reps (60%) / 8 reps (80%)

Repeat both, no rest if possible
Beginner 1 x / Advanced 1 x

CIRCUIT 2
1. Straight Bar Curls 6 reps (80%) / 6- 8 reps (90%)
2. Standing Front Shoulder Press Bar 8 reps (60%) / 6 reps (90%)
3. Plate Front Shoulder Raises 6 reps (10-25lb plate) / 6-8 reps (25lb – 45lb plate)

Repeat all 3, no rest if possible
Beginner 1 x / Advanced 3 x

CIRCUIT 3
1. Standing Curls, dbs. 8 reps (60%) / 6 reps (80%)
2. Alternate Standing Curls, dbs. 10-12 reps (40-50%) / 10-12 Reps (50-70%)

Repeat both, no rest if possible
Beginner NO Repeat / Advanced 2 x

CIRCUIT 4
1. Back, One Arm Rows 10 reps (60%) / 10 reps (70%)
2. Shoulder, Bent Over Raises 10 reps (60%) / 10 reps (70%)

No Repeat

CIRCUIT 5
1. One Arm Row 8 reps (80%) / 5 reps (90%)
2. Bent Over Raises 8 reps (60%) / 6 reps (80%)

Repeat both, no rest if possible
Beginner 2x / Advanced 3x

CIRCUIT 6
1. Back, Low Rows 8 reps (60-70%) / 5 x 5 (95 x 80-90%)
2. Shoulder Side Raises, dbs. 10 reps 50-60% / 6 x 6 (80-90 x 60-70%)
3. Wide Grip Pulls 10-12 (80%) / 8-12 (80-90%)

Repeat all 3, no rest if possible
Beginner 2x / Advanced 4x
Jog 15 minutes

DAY 3

CIRCUIT 1
1. High Knee Jog 5 minutes
2. Mountain Climbers 1 minute
3. Jump Rope 3 minutes
4. Star Jumps 25

Repeat all 3, no rest if possible
Beginner: no repeat / Advanced: 1x

CIRCUIT 2
1. Hanging leg Raises 10 / 20
2. Bicycle 30 sec / 1 min
3. Decline Sit Ups 10 / 20

Repeat all 3, no rest if possible
Beginner: 1x / Advanced: 2-3x

CIRCUIT 3
1. Battle Rope, rope slams 30 reps / 50 reps
2. Dips till failure / till failure * if you're not strong enough try to use a
    gravitron (assisted dips 50% of your weight)
3. Jump Rope 1 min / 1 min

No battle rope? Throw straight punches in air with 1-2 lb dumbbells.
Repeat all 3, no rest if possible
Beginner 1-2x / Advanced 3-4x

DAY 4

CIRCUIT 1
Flat Press, dbs 6-8 reps (70%) / 6-8 reps (80-90%)
Crunches 25 / 50
Repeat both, no rest if possible
Beginner 2 x / Advanced 4 x

CIRCUIT 2
1. Incline Press, dbs 6-8 reps (70%) / 6-8 reps (80-90%)
2. Pull Ups (gravitron or no assistance) till failure / till failure

Repeat both, no rest if possible
Beginner 1x / Advanced 3x

CIRCUIT 3
1. Flat Bench (smith or bar) 15 + reps till failure (50%) / same as beginner but (60-70%)
2. Cable Flies 10 reps (70-80%) / 10-15 reps (80-90%)

Repeat both, no rest if possible
Beginner 0-1x / Advanced 2x

CIRCUIT 4
1. Squat (smith or free bar) 20 reps (50%) / 10 x 15 reps (70% x 50%)
2. Leg Press 20 reps (50-60%) / 10 x 15 reps (80% x 70%)
3. Push Ups *till failure / till failure *drop to knees if can't perform more than 10 reps

Repeat all 3, no rest if possible
Beginner 1x / Advanced 4x

CIRCUIT 5
1. Leg Extension 30 reps (50%) / 30 reps (60-70%)
2. Back Leg Curl 10 reps (60%) / 5 reps x 10 reps (90% x 80%)
3. *Pull Ups till failure / till failure *If using gravitron for assisted

pull ups, set at 50% weight
Repeat all 3, no rest if possible
Beginner 1x / Advanced 2x

DAY 5

CIRCUIT 1
1. Shoulder Press, Bar 5 reps (70%) / 6 reps (80-90%)
2. Shoulder Press, Bar 5 Reps (80%) / 5 reps (70-80%)
3. Straight Bar Curls 10 reps (60%) / 10 reps (70-80%)
4. Straight Bar Curls * (1/2 way) 5 reps / till failure (80%)

*1/2 way rep: bottom to ½ way and back down
Repeat all 3, no rest if possible
Beginner 2x / Advanced 4x

CIRCUIT 2

1. Shoulder, Side to 45 Degrees To Front Raises 5 reps (50%) / 5 reps (70%)
2. Shoulder, Bent Over Raises 10-15 reps (50%) / 10-15 reps (70-80%)
3. Hammer Curls 8-12 reps (60-70%) / 8-12 reps (80-90%)
4. Plate Front Shoulder Raises 6 reps (10-25lb plate) / 6-8 reps (25lb – 45lb plate)

Repeat all 4, no rest if possible
Beginner 2x / Advanced 3x

CIRCUIT 3

1. Upright Row, Bar 10 reps (60-70%) / 10-15 reps (70-80%)
2. Shrugs 10-15 reps (70%) / Shrugs 8-12 reps (80-90%)
3. Close Grip Pulls (back) 6 reps (80%) / 6 reps (90%)
4. Close Grip Pulls 6-10 reps (70%) / 6-10 (80-90%)

Repeat all 4, no rest if possible
Beginner 2x / Advanced 3x

CIRCUIT 4

1. Low Row 6 reps x 6 reps (90% x 70%) / 6 reps x 6-10 reps (90% x 80%)
2. One arm Row 12-15 reps (50%) / 12-15 reps (70%)
3. Leg Raises 25 reps / 50 reps
4. Wide Grip Pulls 15 reps (70%) / 15-20 reps (70-80%)
5. Pull Ups till failure / till failure

Repeat all 5, no rest if possible
Beginner 1x / Advanced 4x

CARDIO
Jog 15-20 minutes

DAY 6

Outside:

Jog
1. mile

Sprints:

Beginner:
- 5 x 25 yard
- 5 x 50 yards
- Jog 1 mile
- Bounding 100 yards and sprint back

Advanced:
- 5 x 25 yard
- 5 x 50 yards
- 2 x 300's
- Jog 2 miles
- 2 x Bounding 100 yards and sprint back

CIRCUIT 1
1. Push Ups 10 reps
2. Sit Ups 10 reps
3. Mountain Climbers 30 sec

Repeat all 3, no rest if possible
Beginner 5x / Advanced 10-20x

DAY 7

Optional but recommended since this program is only 21 days.

CIRCUIT 1
1. Hanging leg raises 20 / 30
2. Bicycle 1 min / 1 min
3. Leg Lifts 10 / 25

4. Plank On Fitness Ball 30 sec / 1 min (roll ball in and out with forearms)

Repeat all 4, no rest if possible
Beginner 2x / Advanced 4x

CIRCUIT 2
1. Jumping Squat w 10-20lb medicine ball 10 reps / 10 reps
2. Stand Ups 20 each leg / 25 each leg
3. Battle Rope, alternate swing 1 min / 1-2 min
4. Pull Ups till failure / till failure
5. Jump Rope 2 min / 3 min

Repeat all 4, no rest if possible
Beginner 1x / Advanced 2-3x

WEEK 2

DAY 8

CIRCUIT 1
1. *Flat Bench Press, bar 8 reps (70%) / 8 reps (70%)
2. Crunches 25 / 50

Repeat both, no rest if possible
Beginner 1x / Advanced 1x
*Perform dumbbells if you have a shoulder problem

CIRCUIT 2
1. Flat Bench Press, bar 5 reps (80%) / 5-6 reps (90%)
2. Leg Lifts 25 / 50

Repeat both, no rest if possible
Beginner 1x, Advanced 2x

CIRCUIT 3
1. Flat Press with *pause 10 reps (60%) / 10 reps (60%)

2. Push Ups 5-10 / 5- till failure

*Pause on chest 2-3 seconds and explode up, hold on top and let down with little resistance. A spotter is most recommended! If you have a spotter, perform till failure at last rep. Perform at own risk and always with a spotter!!
Repeat both, no rest if possible
Beginner 1x / Advanced 2 x

CIRCUIT 4
1. Squat (free bar or smith machine) 10 reps (60%) / 10 reps (70-80%)
2. Back Leg Curls 10-12 reps (80%) / 12-15 reps (70-80%)
3. Jumping Squats 10 / 25 reps holding a 20 lb medicine ball

Repeat all 3, no rest if possible
Beginner 2x / Advanced 2x

CIRCUIT 5 (Advanced Only)
1. Squat (free bar or smith machine) 6-8 reps (80-90% max)
2. Back Leg Curls 8 reps x 12 reps (90% x 80)
3. Overhead Pulls (chest) drop set: 5 reps x 5 reps (95% x 80%)
4. Cable Flies 10 x 10 reps (90 x 80%)
5. Leg Press drop set: 5 reps x 10 reps (90% x 80%)

Repeat all 5, rest 2 min between repeating circuit, stretch after leg press.

Advanced Only 3-4 x
Beginner and Advanced:

CARDIO
Bike, Step Mill or Stair Master 15-20 minutes

DAY 9

CIRCUIT 1
1. Straight Bar Curls 8 reps (80%) / 4 reps x 8 reps (95 x 80%)

2. Standing Front Shoulder Press Bar 5 reps (60-70%) / 5 reps (80-90%)

Repeat both, no rest if possible
Beginner 1x / Advanced 1x

CIRCUIT 2
1. Straight Bar Curls 6 reps (80%) / 6 reps (90%)
2. Standing Curls, dbs (same time) 10 reps (50%) / 10 reps (70%)
3. Standing Front Shoulder Press Bar 8 reps (60%) / 6 reps (90%)
4. Standing Shoulder Press, dbs 10 reps (60%) / 10 reps (60-70%)
5. Battle Rope (alternate) 1 min / 1-2 min
6. Plate Front Shoulder Raises 6 reps (10-25lb plate) / 6-8 reps (25lb – 45lb plate)

Repeat all 6, no rest if possible
Beginner 1x / Advanced 3x

CIRCUIT 3
1. Concentration Curls, dbs 8 reps (60%) / 6 reps (80-90%)
2. Hammer Curls, dbs 10-12 reps (40-50%) / 10-15 Reps (50-70%)

Repeat both, no rest if possible
Beginner NONE / Advanced 2 x

CIRCUIT 4
1. Back, One Arm Row 10 reps (60%) / 10 reps (70%)
2. Shoulder, Bent Over Raises 10 reps (60%) / 10 reps (80-90%)

No Repeat

CIRCUIT 5
1. One Arm Row 8 reps (80%) / 5 reps (95%)
2. Bent over Raises 8 reps (80%) / 6 reps (90%)
3. Shoulder Front Raises-*vertical, dbs 8 reps (60%) / 8 reps (70%)

*place dumbbells on your thighs vertical and lift from thigh to shoulder and repeat.
Repeat all 3, no rest if possible

Beginner 1-2 x / Advanced 3-4 x

CIRCUIT 6
1. Back, Low Rows 8 reps (60-70%) / 5 x 5 (95 x 80-90%)
2. Shoulder Side Raises, dbs. 10 reps 50-60% / 6 x 6 (80-90 x 60-70%)
3. Upright Rows, dbs. 10-12 reps (60-80%) / 6 reps x 6-10 reps (95% x 80-90%)

Repeat all 3, no rest if possible
Beginner 2x / Advanced 4x
Sprint 30 seconds, walk 15 seconds and repeat for 10-15 minutes

DAY 10

CIRCUIT 1
1. Jog 3 minutes, Sprint (90%) 1 minute
2. Mountain Climbers 1 minute
3. Jump Rope 3 minutes
4. Star Jumps 25 / 50

Repeat all 4, no rest if possible
Beginner: 1x / Advanced: 2x

CIRCUIT 2
1. Hanging leg Raises 10 / 20
2. Bicycle 30 sec / 1 min
3. Decline Sit Ups 10 / 25
4. V-Ups 5-10 / 10-20
5. Knee tucks 10 / 25

Repeat all 4, no rest if possible
Beginner 1x / Advanced 2-3x

CIRCUIT 3
1. Battle Rope, slam 50 reps / 50 reps
2. Dips till failure / till failure * if you're not strong enough try to use a Gravitron (assisted dips 50% of your weight)

3. Kettle Bell Swing 1 min / 1 min

Repeat all 3, no rest if possible
Beginner 1-2 x / Advanced 3-4 x

DAY 11

CIRCUIT 1
1. Flat Press, dbs. 6-8 reps (70%) / 6-8 reps (80-90%)
2. Shrugs 10 reps (80%) / 10 reps (80-90%)

Repeat both, no rest if possible
Beginner 2 x / Advanced 4x

CIRCUIT 2
1. Incline Press, dbs. 6-8 reps (70%) / 6-8 reps (80-90%)
2. Close Grip Press, bar 8 reps (60-70%) / 6-8 reps (90%)

Repeat both, no rest if possible
Beginner 1-2x / Advanced 5 x

CIRCUIT 3
1. Tricep Rope Push Downs 15 reps (60-70%) / drop set: 5 x 5 x 5-10 (90 x 80 x 70-80%)
2. Cable flies 10 reps (70%) / drop set: 10 reps x 10 reps (95 x 80-90%)
3. Push Ups till failure / till failure

Repeat both, no rest if possible
Beginner 0-1x / Advanced 3x

CIRCUIT 4
1. Squat (smith or free bar) 15 reps (60-70%) / 6 reps x 10-15 reps (80-90% x 80-70%)
2. Leg Press 20 reps (50-60%) / drop set: 5-8 reps x 10 reps x 10 reps (90% x 80% x 60%)
3. Push Ups *till failure / till failure *drop to knees if can't perform more than 10 reps

Repeat all 3, no rest if possible
Beginner 1x / Advanced 4x

CIRCUIT 5
1. Leg Extension 20 reps (60-70%) / 25 reps (80-90%)
2. Back Leg Curl 10 reps (60%) / 10 reps x 5-8 reps (80% x 70-80%)
3. *Pull Ups till failure / till failure *If using gravitron for assisted pull ups, set at 50% weight

Repeat all 3, no rest if possible
Beginner 1x / Advanced 3x

DAY 12

CIRCUIT 1
1. **Shoulder Press, Bar 5 Reps (80%) / 5 reps (80-90%)
2. Straight Bar Curls 10 reps (70-80%) / 12 reps (80%)
3. Straight Bar Curls * (1/2 way) 5 reps / till failure

*1/2 way rep: bottom to ½ way and back down
4. Shoulder press, dbs. 5 reps (70%) / 5-8 reps (70%)
5. Push Ups, feet up on elevation 3-5 inches 5 reps / 10 reps

** Warm Up Shoulders with light weight
Repeat all 5, no rest if possible
Beginner 2x / Advanced 4x

CIRCUIT 2
1. Shoulder, Side to 45 Degrees To Front Raises 5 reps (50%) / 5 reps (70%)
2. Shoulder, Bent Over Raises 10-15 reps (50%) / 10-15 reps (60%)
3. Hammer Curls 8-12 reps (60-70%) / 8-12 reps (80-90%)

Repeat all 3, no rest if possible
Beginner 2x / Advanced 3x

CIRCUIT 3
1. Upright Row, Bar 10 reps (60-70%) / 10-15 reps (70-80%)

2. Shrugs 10-15 reps (70%) / Shrugs 8-12 reps (80-90%)
3. Back-Close Grip Pulls 6-8 reps (90%) / 6 x 6-10 reps (90 x 80-90%)
4. Chin Up Hold: Hold chin over bar as long as you can for 1 rep
5. Wide Grip Pull Down 6 reps (90%) / 6 -8 reps (90%)

Repeat all 5, no rest if possible
Beginner 2x / Advanced 3x

CIRCUIT 4

1. Low Row 5 x 5 reps (80%- 70-80%) / 5 x 5-10 (90% x 80-90%)
2. One arm Row 10-15 reps (50-70%) / 10-15 reps (60-80%)
3. Plank 1 min / 1min
4. Wide Grip Pulls 5 reps (8-90%) / 5 reps (80-90%)
5. Crunches 25 / 50

Repeat all 5, no rest if possible
Beginner 2-3x / Advanced 4 x

CARDIO
Jog 20-30 minutes

DAY 13

Outside:
Jog
1. mile

Sprints:
Beginner:
- 5 x 25 yard
- 5 x 50 yards
- Jog 1 mile
- 2 x Bound 100 yards, sprint back to finish

Advanced:
- 5 x 25 yard
- 5 x 50 yards

- 2 x 300's
- Jog 2 miles
- 3 x Bound 100 yards and sprint back to finish

CIRCUIT 1
1. Push Ups 10
2. Sit Ups 10
3. Mountain Climbers 30 sec

Repeat all 3, no rest if possible
Beginner 5-10 x / Advanced 10-20x

DAY 14

CIRCUIT 1
1. Hanging leg raises 20 / 30
2. Bicycle 1 min / 1 min
3. Leg Lifts 10 / 25
4. Plank On Fitness Ball 30 sec / 1 min (roll ball in and out with arms)
5. Knee Tucks 10 / 25

Repeat all 4, no rest if possible
Beginner 2x / Advanced 4x

CIRCUIT 2
1. Jumping Squat w 10-20 lb. medicine ball 10 reps / 10 reps
2. Battle Rope, alternate 1 min / 1-2 min
3. Pull Ups till failure / till failure
4. Stand Ups 25 each leg / 25 each leg
5. Jump Rope 2 min / 3 min
6. Kettle Bell 1 min / 2 min

Repeat all 6, no rest if possible
Beginner 1-2 x / Advanced 3-4 x

WEEK 3

DAY 15

CIRCUIT 1
1. *Flat Bench Press, bar 8 reps (70%) / 8 reps (70%)
2. Crunches 25 / 50
3. Hanging Leg Raises 10 / 30

Repeat all 3, no rest if possible
Beginner 1 x / Advanced 1 x
*Perform dumbbells if you have a shoulder problem

CIRCUIT 2
1. Flat Bench Press 5 reps x 5 reps (80 x 70%) / drop set 3-6 reps x
   5-8 reps (95% x 70-80%)
2. Leg Lifts 25 / 25

Repeat all 2, no rest if possible
Beginner 1 x, Advanced 3 x

CIRCUIT 3
1. Flat Press with *pause 6 reps (70%) / 8 reps (70%)
2. Shrugs 15 reps (70%) / 12 – 15 reps (80%)

*Pause on chest 2-3 seconds and explode up, hold on top and let
down with little resistance. A spotter is most recommended! If you
have a spotter, perform till failure at last rep. Perform at own risk!!
Repeat both, no rest if possible
Beginner 2 x / Advanced 3-4 x

CIRCUIT 4
1. Squat (free bar or smith machine) 8 reps (70%) / 6 reps (80%)
2. Back Leg Curls 10 reps (70-80%) / 10-15 reps (80-90%)
3. Alternate Lunges 10 each leg (80%) / 6 each leg (90%)
4. Good Mornings 10 / 10

Repeat all 4, no rest if possible
Beginner 2 x / Advanced 4 x

CIRCUIT 5

Advanced Only
1. Squat (free bar or smith machine) Advanced only 20 reps (60-70% max)
2. Overhead Pulls (chest) 5 reps x 5 reps x 5 reps (95% x 90% x 80%)
3. Cable Flies 10 reps (80-90%)
4. Leg Press 5 x 10 reps x 5 reps (90% x 80% x 70-80%)

Repeat all 4, rest 2 min between repeating circuit, stretch after leg press.

Advanced Only 4 x

CARDIO
Bike, Step Mill or Stair Master 15-20 minutes

DAY 16

CIRCUIT 1
1. Straight Bar Curls 8 reps (80%) / 6 reps (80%)
2. Standing Front Shoulder Press Bar 5 reps (60-70%) / 5 reps (80-90%)

No repeat

CIRCUIT 2
1. Straight Bar Curls 6 reps (80%) / 6 reps (90%)
2. Cable Curls with straight bar till failure (80%) / till failure (80%)
3. Standing Front Shoulder Press Bar 6 reps (60%) / 6 reps (90%)
4. Upright rows, dbs 10 reps (70%) / 5 x 5 x 5 (90 x 80 x 70-80%)
5. Plate Front Shoulder Raises 6 reps (10-25lb plate) / 6-8 reps (25lb – 45lb plate)

Repeat all 5, no rest if possible
Beginner 2 x / Advanced 4 x

CIRCUIT 3
1. Concentration Curls, dbs 8 reps (60%) / 6 reps (80-90%)
2. Hammer Curls, dbs 10-12 reps (40-50%) / 10-15 Reps (60-70%)
3. Shoulder Front raise w plate 8 reps (10-25lb) / 8 reps (35-45lb)

Repeat all 3, no rest if possible
Beginner 2 x / Advanced 2 x

CIRCUIT 4
1. Back, One Arm Row 10 reps (60%) / 10 reps (70%)
2. Shoulder, Bent Over Raises 10 reps (60%) / 10 reps (70%)

No Repeat

CIRCUIT 5
1. One Arm Row 5 reps (80%) / 5 reps (90%)
2. Bent Over Raises 8 reps (60%) / 3-5 reps x 5-8 reps (90 x 80%)
3. One Arm Row 10 reps (70%) / 8 reps (70%)
4. Shoulder Front Raises-regular, dbs. 8 reps (60%) / 8 reps (70%)
5. Cable curls, small bar 20-30 reps (50-60%) / 20-40 reps (70-80%)

Repeat all 5, no rest if possible
Beginner 1 x / Advanced 4 x

CIRCUIT 6
1. Back, Low Rows 8 reps (60-70%) / 5 x 5-10 (95 x 80-90%)
2. Shoulder Side Raises, dbs. 10 reps (80%) / 6 x 6 (90 x 70-80%)
3. V- Grip Pull Down, v-bar (back) 8-10 reps (80%) / 8-10 reps (80-90%) at end of 10 reps: pulse from chest to 5-6 inches for another 8-12 reps.

Repeat all 3, no rest if possible
Beginner 3 x / Advanced 4 x
Jog 15 minutes

DAY 17

CIRCUIT 1
1. Jog 3 minutes, Sprint (70%) 1 minute
2. Mountain Climbers 1 minute
3. Jump Rope 3 minutes

Repeat all 3, no rest if possible
Beginner: 1 x / Advanced: 2 x

CIRCUIT 2
1. Hanging leg Raises 15 / 30
2. Bicycle 30 sec / 1 min
3. Decline Sit Ups 15-20 / 30
4. V-Ups 5-10 / 10-20

Repeat all 4, no rest if possible
Beginner 0-1 x / Advanced 2-3 x

CIRCUIT 3
1. Battle Rope 30 sec / 1 min
2. Dips till failure / till failure * if you're not strong enough try to use a gravitron (assisted dips 50% of your weight)
3. Kettle Bell 1 min / 2 min
4. Rope 1 min / 2 min

Repeat all 4, no rest if possible
Beginner 0-1 x / Advanced 2-3 x
Jog
1-2 miles

DAY 18

CIRCUIT 1
1. Flat Press, dbs 6-8 reps (70%) / 6-8 reps (80-90%)
2. Plank 1 min / 2 min

Repeat both, no rest if possible

Beginner 2 x / Advanced 4x

CIRCUIT 2
1. Incline Press, dbs. 6-8 reps (70%) / 6-8 reps (80-90%)
2. Close Grip Press, bar 8 reps (80%) / 8 reps (90%)

Repeat both, no rest if possible
Beginner 2x / Advanced 4x

CIRCUIT 3
1. Tricep Rope Push Downs 15-25 reps (60-70%) / 5 x 5 x 5-10 (90 x 80 x 70-80%)
2. Cable flies 10 reps - 15 (70%) / 10 – 15 reps (90%)

Repeat both, no rest if possible
Beginner 1x / Advanced 3x

CIRCUIT 4
1. Squat (smith or free bar) 15 reps (60-70%) / 10 x 10 (90% x 80-90%)
2. Leg Press 20 reps (50-60%) / 5-8 x 10 x 10 (90% x 80-90% x 60-70%)
3. Overhead Tricep 20 reps (80%) / 20 Reps (80%)
4. Dips till failure / till failure
5. Tricep Push Ups till failure / till failure

Repeat all 5, no rest if possible
Beginner 2 x / Advanced 3-4 x

CIRCUIT 5
1. Front Squat w db 10 reps (80%) / 10-15 reps (80%)
2. Leg Extension 20 reps (60-70%) / 25 reps (70-80%)
3. Back Leg Curl 10 reps (60%) / 5 reps x 10 reps (90% x 80%)
4. Lunges 15 each side / 10 each side holding 10-25lbs each hand

Repeat all 4, no rest if possible
Beginner 1-2 x / Advanced 3 x

DAY 19

CIRCUIT 1
1. *Shoulder Press, Bar 5 Reps (80%) / 5 reps (80-90%)
2. Straight Bar Curls 10 reps (70-8%) / 10 reps (80-90%)
3. Straight Bar Curls * (1/2 way) 5 reps / till failure
      *1/2 way rep: bottom to ½ way and back down
4. Push Ups, feet up on elevation 3-5 inches 5 reps / 10 reps

*Warm Up Shoulders with light weight
Repeat all 3, no rest if possible
Beginner 2 x / Advanced 4 x

CIRCUIT 2
1. Shoulder, Side to 45 Degrees To Front Raises 5 reps (50%) / 5
      reps (80%)
2. Shoulder, Bent Over Raises 10-15 reps (50%) / 6 reps (90%)
3. Shoulder, Bent Over Raises (Advanced only) till failure 70-80%
4. Plate Front Shoulder Raises 6 reps (10-25lb plate) / 6-8 reps (25lb
      – 45lb plate)
5. Hammer Curls 8-12 reps (60-70%) / 8-12 reps (80-90%)

Repeat all 5, no rest if possible
Beginner 2 x / Advanced 4 x

CIRCUIT 3
1. Upright Row, Bar 10 reps (60-70%) / 10-15 resp (70-80%)
2. Shrugs 10-15 reps (70%) / Shrugs 8-12 reps (80-90%)
3. Back-Close Grip Pulls 6 reps (80%) / 6 reps (90%)
4. Back-Wide Grip Pulls 6-10 reps (70-80%) / 6-10 (80-90%)
5. Chin Up: Hold chin over bar as long as you can for 1 rep

Repeat all 5, no rest if possible
Beginner 2x / Advanced 4 x

CIRCUIT 4
1. Low Row 6 reps (80%) / 6 reps (90%)
2. Low Row 6-10 reps (70-80%) / 6-10 reps (80-90%)

3. One arm Row 12-15 reps (50%) / 12-15 reps (60%)

Repeat all 3, no rest if possible
Beginner 1 x / Advanced 3x

CARDIO
Jog 20-30 minutes

DAY 20

Outside:

Jog
1. mile

Sprints:
Beginner:
- 5 x 25 yard
- 5 x 50 yards
- Jog 1-2 mile
- 2-3 x Bound 100 yards and sprint back to starting line.

Advanced:
- 5 x 25 yard
- 5 x 50 yards
- 2 x 300's
- Jog 2-3 miles
- 3-4 x Bound 100 yards and sprint back to starting line.

CIRCUIT 1
1. Push Ups 10
2. Sit Ups 10
3. Mountain Climbers 30 sec

Repeat all 3, no rest if possible
Beginner 5-10x / Advanced 15-20x
Jog
1. mile

DAY 21

CIRCUIT 1
1. Hanging leg raises 20 / 30
2. Bicycle 1 min / 1 min
3. Leg Lifts 25 / 50
4. Plank On Fitness Ball 30 sec / 1 min (roll ball in and out with arms)

Repeat all 4, no rest if possible
Beginner 3x / Advanced 5x

CIRCUIT 2
1. Jumping Squat w 10-20lb medicine ball 10 reps / 15 reps
2. Battle Rope 1 min / 1-2 min
3. Pull Ups till failure / till failure
4. Chin Ups till failure / till failure
5. Jump Rope 2 min / 3 min

Repeat all 5, no rest if possible
Beginner 1-2 x / Advanced 3 x

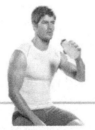

GUY #3
SPORTS GUY

OK there champ. Time for you to go from a slob to fit. Let's get you back into fighting shape. Faster, leaner and a shit load of more confidence.

Don't keep looking at your past saying how fit you once were when in high school or college. Do something about it.

The key goal with this program: to increase muscle and cardio endurance. In 3 weeks, I'm hoping you'll enjoy sweating, running and feeling lighter.

No. You're not going to do just burpees and mountain climbers like every other jack ass, copycat training program from these wannabe trainers.

PHASE 2

DAY 1

Beginner
Jog 1 mile (if you can't jog a mile then walk and trot)

Advanced
Jog 2 miles (every 2 minutes pick up the pace 80% for 30 seconds)

CIRCUIT 1
1. Push Ups 10-20 / 30-50
2. High Plank 1 min / 2 min
3. Back N' Forth 1 min / 2 min
4. Pull Ups 30 sec jumping / 30 sec jumping
5. Chin Ups 15 sec jumping / 30 sec jumping
6. Chin Up with Hold till failure / till failure (hold your chin over bar)

Repeat all 6, no rest if possible
Beginner 1-2 x / Advanced 3-4 x

CARDIO:
Boxing: 10 Punch Drill x 10
Jumping Squat 20 / 50

DAY 2

CIRCUIT 1
1. Jump Rope 2 min / 3 min
2. Bosu Lateral X-Over 1 min / 2 min or Back N Forth if you don't have a bosu.
3. Jumping Squat 30 sec / 1 min

Repeat all 3, no rest if possible
Beginner 2 x / Advanced 3 x

Warm Up
1. Straight Bar Curls 10 (60%) / 10 (70%)
2. Front Shoulder Press, Bar 10 (60%) / 10 (70%)
3. Squats Free Bar, Smith Machine or Db 12 (60%) / 12 (60%)

CIRCUIT 2
1. Straight Bar Curls 5 reps (70-80%) / 5 reps (80-90%)
2. Straight Bar Curls 5-8 reps (60-70%) / 10 reps (70-80%)
3. Front Shoulder Press, Bar 5 reps (70-80%) / 5 reps (80-90%)
4. Front Shoulder Press, Bar 5-8 reps (60-70%) / 8-10 reps (70-80%)
5. Squats Free Bar, Smith Machine or Db 12 reps (60-70%) / 10 (70-80%)

Repeat all 5, no rest if possible
Beginner 1-3 x / Advanced 2-4x
1. Jumping Jacks with a fist 2 min / 3 min
2. Burpees 10 / 30
3. Jumping Squats 10 / 25
4. Wall sit 30 sec / 1-2 minutes
5. Bosu X-Over 1-2 minutes

Sign up to get Exercise Clips and workout videos
www.fitactions.com/builditworkoutvideos

DAY 3

Cardio

Beginner:
Jog 1 mile

Sprints (70% max intensity):
- 5 x 25 yards, rest with walk back
- 3 x 50 yards, rest with walk back
- Bounding 2 x 25 yards, sprint back to starting line
- Power Skips 2 x 25 yards
- Back N' Forth 1 min

Jog 1 mile
Boxing: 10 Punch Drill x 10

Advanced:
Jog 1 mile

Sprints (70% max intensity):
- 5 x 25 yards, rest with walk back
- 3 x 50 yards, rest with walk back
- 300 (sprint 80% from starting line to 50 yards and back, repeat 6x = 300 yards) no rest. Time yourself for future reference.
- Bounding 2 x 50 yards, sprint back to starting line
- Power Skips 2 x 50 yards
- Back N Forth 1 min

Bleachers or Hill sprints 3 x 3 minutes (sprint up a hill 25-50 yards, trot down)
Boxing: 10 Punch Drill x 10

DAY 4

Bike or Jog 10 minutes

CIRCUIT 1

1. Flat Bench Press, bar or db 15 reps (60%) / 15 reps (70%)
2. One Arm Row 15 reps (60%) / 20 reps(60%)
3. Battle Rope, Alternate 1 min / 2 min

Repeat both:
Beginner 1 x / Advanced 1 x

CIRCUIT 2
1. Bench Press, bar or db 10 reps (70%) / 10 reps (80-90%)
2. One Arm Row 12 reps (70-80%) / 8 reps (80-90%)
3. Pull Ups Jumping 30 sec / 30 sec
4. Jump Rope 1 min / 1 min

Repeat all 4, No rest if possible
Beginner 2 x / Advanced 4 x

CIRCUIT 3
1. Tricep Close Grip Press Bar 10 reps (60%) / 10 Reps (80%)
2. Burpees 10 / 20
3. Hanging Leg Raises 15 / 30

Repeat all 3, no rest if possible
Beginner 1-2 x / Advanced 2-3 x

CIRCUIT 4
1. Push ups 5
2. Heavy Bag Punches 20 (hard punches)

Repeat both, 5-10 x

DAY 5

CARDIO

Beginner:

Jog 2 miles
Jump Rope 3 minutes

Boxing: 10 Punch Drill x 10

CIRCUIT 1
1. Squat, dumbbell 20 reps 50-60% max
2. Plank 1-2 minutes
3. Upright Rows, bar or dbs 10 reps (70%)
4. Wall sit 30 seconds

Repeat all 4, no rest if possible, 2-4 x

Advanced:

Jog 2-3 miles
Jump Rope 3 minutes
Boxing: 10 Punch Drill x 10

CIRCUIT 1
1. Squat, dumbbell 20 reps (70-80%)
2. Plank 1-2 minutes
3. Dead Lifts 6 reps (60 - 70%)
4. Upright rows, bar or db 10 reps (80-90%)
5. Jump Rope 1 min
6. Bosu X-Over or Skating if no Bosu 2 minutes

Repeat all 6, no rest if possible, 3-5 x

DAY 6

Warm Up
1. Jump Rope 1 min / 1 min
2. Front Shoulder Press, Bar 10 reps (50%) / 10 reps (50%)
3. Standing Curls, bar 10 reps (50%) / 10 reps (50%)
4. Battle Rope (alternate) 1 min / 1 min

CIRCUIT 1
1. Jump Rope 1 min / 1 min
2. Front Shoulder Press, Bar 8 reps (60%) / 8 reps (70-90%)
3. Standing Curls, Bar 5- 8 reps (70-80%) / 5 reps (80-90%)

4. Battle Rope (2 arm slam) 25 reps / 50 reps

Repeat all 4, no rest if possible
Beginner 3-4 x / Advanced 4-5 x

3-Rounds: Heavy Bag (Level 1) 3 minute Rounds
In-between rounds: 25 body weight squats, 10 push-ups, 30 sec. Jump Rope

DAY 7

Rest or Jog

If Jogging:
Beginner: Trot Jog 2-3 miles

Advanced: Jog 4-6 miles

WEEK 2

DAY 8

Beginner
Jog 1 mile
Stretch Hamstrings, Back and Quads 5-10 min
Sprint (80%) 3 x 25 yards or 3 x 30 seconds

Advanced
Jog 2 miles (every 2 minutes pick up the pace 80% for 30 seconds)
Stretch Hamstrings, Back and Quads 5-10 min
Sprint (80%) 5 x 25 or 5 x 30 seconds

CIRCUIT 1
1. Flat Bench Press, Bar or Dumbbell 10 Reps (70%) / 10 reps (80%)
2. Push Ups 5-10 reps / 10-20 reps
3. High Plank 30 seconds / 1 minute
4. Mountain Climbers 30 seconds / 1 Minute

Repeat all 4, no rest if possible
Beginner 2 x / Advanced 4 x

CIRCUIT 2
1. Pull Ups 30 sec jumping / 30 sec jumping
2. Chin Ups 15 sec jumping / 30 sec jumping
3. Chin Up with Hold till failure / till failure (hold your chin over bar)
4. Kettle Bell Swing 1 min / 2 min
5. Battle Rope (alternate) 30 sec / 1 min

Repeat all 5, no rest if possible
Beginner 2-3 x / Advanced 4-5 x

CARDIO:
1. Boxing: 10 Punch Drill
2. Sit Ups 50
3. Heavy Bag Hooks 50 each side

Repeat all 3, 3x

DAY 9

CIRCUIT 1
1. Jump Rope 2 min / 3 min
2. *Bosu or Box Lateral X-Over 1 min / 2 min
3. Mountain Climbers 30 sec / 1 min
4. **Alternate Layups 1 min / 1 min

*skate if you don't have a Bosu or a 12-16 inch box.
**Power Skip in place alternating legs, reaching up as if doing a layup in basketball

Repeat all 3, no rest if possible
Beginner 1 x / Advanced 1 x

CIRCUIT 1
1. Straight Bar Curls 12 (60%) / 12-15 (70%)
2. Front Shoulder Press, Bar 10 (60%) / 10-12 (70-80%)

3. Squats Free Bar, Smith Machine or Db 15 (60%) / 15 (60%)

No Repeat

CIRCUIT 2
1. Straight Bar Curls 5 reps (70-80%) / 5 reps (80-90%)
2. Straight Bar Curls 5-8 reps (60-70%) / 10 reps (70-80%)
3. Squat and Press dbs., shoulder 6 reps (10-15lbs) / 6 – 8 reps (15-30lbs)
4. Front Shoulder Press, Bar 5-8 reps (60-70%) / 8-10 reps (70-80%)
5. Squats Free Bar, Smith Machine or Db 5 (70-80%) / 6 (80-90%)
6. Squats Free Bar, Smith Machine or Db 10 (50-60%) / 10 (60-80%)

Repeat all 6, no rest if possible
Beginner 2 x / Advanced 3-4 x

CIRCUIT 3
1. Jumping Jacks with a fist or Jump Rope 2 min / 3 min
2. Star Jumps 25 / 50
3. Jumping Squats 25 / 50
4. Push Ups till failure / till failure
5. Skating 1 min / 1min

No Repeat

Sign up to get Exercise Clips and workout videos
www.fitactions.com/builditworkoutvideos

DAY 10

Cardio

Beginner:
Jog 1 mile

Sprints (70% max intensity):
- 5 x 25 yards, rest with trot back
- 3 x 50 yards, rest with walk back

- 2 x 100 yards, rest with walk back
- Bounding 2 x 50 yards, sprint back to starting line.
- Power Skips 1 x 50 yards
- Back N' Forth 3 x 1 min, 15 sec rest in between each minute

Jog 1 mile

Boxing: 10 Punch Drill x 10

Advanced:
Jog 1 mile

Sprints (70% max intensity):
- 5 x 25 yards, rest with trot back
- 3 x 50 yards, rest with walk back
- 300 (jog start line to 50 yards and back, repeat 6x = 300 yards) no rest. Time yourself for future reference.
- Bounding 3 x 50 yards, sprint back to starting line.
- Power Skips 3 x 50 yards, rest by trotting back to starting line
- Back N' Forth 3 x 1 min, 15 sec rest in between each minute

Jog 3-4 miles
Boxing: 10 Punch Drill x 10

DAY 11

Bike or Jog 10 minutes

CIRCUIT 1
Flat Chest Press, bar or db 15 reps (60%) / 15 reps (70%)
Incline Chest Press, bar or db 10 reps (60%) / 10 reps (60%)
One Arm Row 15 reps (60%) / 20 reps (60%)

No Repeat

CIRCUIT 2
1. Flat Chest Press, bar or db 8 reps (70%) / 6 reps (80-90%)
2. One Arm Row 12 reps (70-80%) / 8 reps (80-90%)

3. Push Ups 5 / 5-10
4. Pull Ups Jumping 30 sec / 30 sec
5. Jump Rope 1 min / 1 min

Repeat all 5, No rest if possible
Beginner 2 x / Advanced 3 x

CIRCUIT 3
1. Incline Chest Press, bar or db 10 reps (60%) / 10 reps (70-80%)
2. Tricep Close Grip Bar 10 reps (60%) / 10 Reps (80%)
3. Gym: Wide Grip Pull Down or Home: Pull Ups 10 (80%) / 10 (80-90%)
4. Hanging Leg Raises 15 / 30
5. Decline Sit Ups 10-15 / 20-30

Repeat all 5, no rest if possible
Beginner 1-2 x / Advanced 3-4 x

DAY 12

CARDIO

Beginner:

Jog 1 mile
Jump Rope 3 minutes
Battle Rope (rope slams) 50 reps / 100 reps
Boxing: 10 Punch Drill x 10

CIRCUIT 1
1. Squat, bar or dumbbell 10 reps (50-60%)
2. Squat, bar or dumbbell 10 reps (60-70%)
3. Kettle Bell or Db Swings 1 min 10-15lbs
4. Plank 1-2 minutes
5. Leg Lifts 10-25
6. Upright Rows, bar or dbs 10 reps (70%)
7. Shrugs 15 reps (80%)
8. Push-ups or Dips Till Failure

Repeat all 8, no rest if possible, 3-4 x

Advanced:

Jog 2 miles
Jump Rope 3 minutes
Boxing: 10 Punch Drill x 10

CIRCUIT 1
1. Squat, db 5 reps (90%)
2. Squat, bar or dumbbell 15 reps (60-70%)
3. Kettle Bell or Db Swings 1 min 10-25 lbs
4. Dead Lifts, bar or db 8 reps (70-80%)
5. Leg Lifts (abs) 10-25
6. Upright Rows, bar or dbs 10 reps (80-90%)
7. Shrugs 15 reps (80%)
8. Dips Till Failure

Repeat all 8, no rest if possible, 3-5 x

DAY 13

Warm Up
1. Jump Rope 1 min
2. Front Shoulder Press, Bar 10 reps (50%) / 10 reps (50%)
3. Standing Curls, bar 10 reps (50%) / 10 reps (50%)

CIRCUIT 1
1. Jump Rope 1 min
2. Front Shoulder Press, Bar 8 reps (70%) / 8 reps (80-90%)
3. Standing Curls, Bar 5- 8 reps (70-80%) / 5 reps (80-90%)
4. Chin Ups Till Failure / Till Failure
5. Pull Ups Till Failure / Till Failure

Repeat all 3, no rest if possible
Beginner 3-4 x / Advanced 4-5 x

CIRCUIT 2

3-Rounds Boxing (Level 1) Heavy Bag 3 minute rounds
Active Rest (in-between rounds peform all 4 exercises below):
1. Jump Rope 30 sec
2. Back N' Forth 30 Sec
3. Push Ups 10
4. Bosu X Over 1 min

Repeat 3 min boxing rounds, 3x

Optional:
Bike or Jog 1-4 miles

DAY 14

Rest (hmm. Its only 3 weeks!) Or Jog
If Running:
Beginner: Jog 3 miles

Advanced: Jog 5-6 miles

WEEK 3

DAY 15

Beginner
Jog 1 mile (if you can't jog a mile then walk and trot)
Sprint (90%) 5 x 25 yards or 5 x 30 seconds

Advanced
Jog 2 miles (every 2 minutes pick up the pace 80% for 30 seconds)
Sprint (90%) 5 x 25 or 5 x 30 seconds, 5 x 50 yards or 5 x 45 sec

CIRCUIT 1
1. Flat Bench Press, Bar or Dumbbell 8 Reps (80%) / 6 reps (90%)
2. Push Ups 5-10 reps / 10-20 reps
3. High Plank 1 minute / 2 minutes
4. Mountain Climbers 30 seconds / 1 Minute

5. Jump Rope 1 min / 1 min
6. Star Jumps 25 / 50

Repeat all 6, no rest if possible
Beginner 2 x / Advanced 4 x

CIRCUIT 2
1. Gym: Close Grip Pulls 30 reps (50%) / 30 reps (60%) or Home: One Arm Row 15 reps each arm (60%) and chin ups till failure / till failure
2. Dips till failure / till failure
3. Pull Ups 30 sec jumping / 30 sec jumping
4. Chin Ups 15 sec jumping / 30 sec jumping
5. Chin Up with Hold till failure / till failure (hold your chin over bar)

Repeat all 5, no rest if possible
Beginner 2-3 x / Advanced 4-5 x

CARDIO:

Boxing: 10 Punch Drill x 10
1. Push Ups 50
2. Straight Bag Punches 100
3. Hooks To Bag, head 100
4. Shovel Punch to Bag, body 100

DAY 16

CIRCUIT 1
1. Jump Rope 2 min / 3 min
2. Bosu or Box Lateral X-Over 1 min / 2 min
3. Mountain Climbers 1 min / 2 min

*skate if you don't have a Bosu or Box
Repeat all 3, no rest if possible
Beginner 1 x / Advanced 1 x

Warm Up

CIRCUIT 1
1. Straight Bar Curls 12 (60%) / 12 (70%)
2. Front Shoulder Press, Bar 10 (60%) / 10 (70%)
3. Squats Free Bar, Smith Machine or Db 15 (60%) / 15 (70%)

No Repeat

CIRCUIT 2
1. Straight Bar Curls 5 x 5-8 reps (90 x 80%) / 5 x 10 reps (90 x 80%)
2. Standing Hammer Curls 10 reps (70%) / 10 reps (80%)
3. Front Shoulder Press, Bar 5 x 5 reps (80 x 70%) / 5 x 5 reps (90 x 80%)
4. Shoulder Press, Standing db. 5 reps (70%) / 5 reps (70-80%)
5. Squats Free Bar, Smith Machine or Db 5 x 10 reps (90 x 80%) / 6 x 10 reps (90 x 80%)

Repeat all 5, no rest if possible
Beginner 2 x / Advanced 3-4 x

CIRCUIT 3
1. Jumping Jacks with a fist or Jump Rope 2 min / 3 min
2. Jumping Squat with a weight (medicine ball or db) 10 / 20
3. Star Jumps 25 / 50

Sign up to get Exercise Clips and workout videos
www.fitactions.com/builditworkoutvideos

DAY 17

Cardio

Beginner:

Jog 1 mile

Sprints (70% max intensity):
- 5 x 25 yards, rest with trot back
- 5 x 50 yards, rest with trot back

- 2 x 100 yards, rest with walk back
- Bounding 3 x 100 yards, jog back to starting line.
- Power Skips 1 x 100 yards
- Back N' Forth 3-4 x 1 min, 15 sec rest in between each minute

Bleachers or Hill sprints (sprint up 25-50 feet and trot back down)
-2 x 3 minute

Jog 1-2 miles

Advanced:

Jog 1 mile

Sprints (100% max intensity):
- 2 x 300 (jog start line to 50 yards and back, repeat 6x = 300 yards) no rest. Time yourself
- 5 x 25 yards, rest with trot back
- 3 x 50 yards, rest with walk back
- 3x 100 yards, rest with walk back
- Bounding 2 x 100 yards, sprint back to starting line.
- Power Skips 4 x 100 yards, 30 sec rest between
- Back N' Forth 3-5 x 1 min, 15 sec rest in between each minute

Bleachers or Hill (sprint up 25-50 feet and trot back down) sprints
-3 x 3 min

Jog 2-3 miles

DAY 18

Bike or Jog 10 minutes

CIRCUIT 1
1. Flat Chest Press, bar or db. 15 reps (60%) / 15 reps (70%)
2. Incline Chest Press, bar or db. 10 reps (60%) / 10 reps (60%)
3. One Arm Row 15 reps (60%) / 20 reps (60%)

CIRCUIT 2
1. Flat Chest Press, bar or db 8 reps (80%) / 4-6 reps (90-95%)
2. One Arm Row 12 reps (80%) / 6-8 reps (80-95%)
3. Push Ups 5 / 5-10
4. Pull Ups Jumping 30 sec / 1 min
5. Jump Rope 1 min / 1 min
6. Battle Rope (rope slams) 50 reps / 50 reps
7. Battle Rope (alternate) 30 sec - 1 min / 1 min

Repeat all 7, No rest if possible
Beginner 2-3 x / Advanced 3-4 x

CIRCUIT 3
1. Incline Chest Press, bar or db. 10 reps (70-80%) / 6 reps (80-90%)
2. Tricep Close Grip Bar 6 reps (60-70%) / 6 Reps (80%)
3. Wide Grip Pull Down (Gym) or Pull Ups 8 reps (80%) / 10 reps (80-90%)
4. Close Grip Pulls Down (Gym) or Chin Ups 5 reps (90%) / 5 reps (90%)
5. Hanging Leg Raises 15 / 30
6. Decline Sit Ups 10-15 / 20-30
7. High Plank 30 sec – 1min / plank 1 min

Repeat all 7, no rest if possible
Beginner 1-2 x / Advanced 3-4 x

DAY 19

CARDIO

Beginner:

Jog 1 mile
Jump Rope 3 minutes
3 – 3 minute Heavy Bag Workout (level 1)

CIRCUIT 1
1. Squat, bar or dumbbell 10 reps (70 %)

2. Squat, bar or dumbbell 10 reps (60-70%)
3. Kettle Bell or Db Swings 1 min 10-15lbs
4. Jump and Squat 25
5. Plank 1-2 minutes
6. Leg Lifts 10-25
7. Upright Rows, bar or dbs. 10 reps (70%)
8. Shrugs 15 reps (80%)
9. Pushups or Dips Till Failure

Repeat all 9, no rest if possible, 2-4 x

Advanced:

Jog 1 mile
Jump Rope 3 minutes
5 – 3 minute Heavy Bag Workout (level 1)

CIRCUIT 1
1. Squat, dumbbell 5 reps (90%)
2. Squat, bar or dumbbell 15 reps (70-80%)
3. Kettle Bell or Db Swings 1 min 10-15lbs
4. Dead Lifts, bar or db. 8 reps (70-80%)
5. Leg Lifts 10-25
6. Jump and Squat Holding 10-25 lb. medicine ball 25 reps
7. Upright Rows, bar or dbs. 10 reps (80-90%)
8. Shrugs 15 reps (80%)
9. Rope (alternate) 1 min / 1min
10. Dips Till Failure

Repeat all 10, no rest if possible, 3-5 x

DAY 20

Warm Up
1. Jump Rope 1 min
2. Front Shoulder Press, Bar 10 reps (50%) / 10 reps (50%)
3. Standing Curls, bar 10 reps (50%) / 10 reps (50%)

CIRCUIT 1
1. Jump Rope 1 min
2. Front Shoulder Press, bar 5-6 reps (80%) / 4-6 reps (90%)
3. Standing Curls, bar 5-8 reps (70-80%) / 5-8 reps (80-90%)
4. Chin Ups Till Failure / Till Failure
5. Pull Ups Till Failure / Till Failure

Repeat all 3, no rest if possible
Beginner 3-4x / Advanced 5x

CIRCUIT 2
4-Rounds Boxing (Level 1) Heavy Bag 3 minute rounds
Active Rest (in-between rounds perform all 4 exercises):
1. Jump Rope 30 sec
2. Back N' Forth 30 Sec
3. Push Ups 10
4. Skate 1 min

Optional:
Bike or Jog 1-4 miles

DAY 21

Rest (hmm. Its only 3 weeks!) or Jog

Beginner: Jog 3-4 miles
Advanced: Jog 6-8 miles

YOU did it! Well, I hope you did. You should feel absolutely more fit and stronger. Now, I recommend trying the Guy #2 program and then going back to this program for the 3rd session.

EXERCISE DESCRIPTIONS AND PICTORIALS

Below are all the exercises shown briefly on the correct form and execution. For a live view of exercises and workouts. Sign up for FREE Bonus Videos and workouts at
www.fitactions/builditworkoutvideos

CHEST EXERCISES

Chest Press (dumbbells):

- Start from top extended position. Lower slowly. Elbows should go parallel to bench, stretching chest. Squeeze pecs and press up with force.
- Hold on top 2 seconds and repeat. Feet flat on floor or on bench (advanced only).

Primary Lift: builds mass and strength.

Pros: only use dumbbells for chest press if you have had a rotator or shoulder injury in the past. Heavy dumbbell helps build your chest. Dumbbells are also great for helping develop muscle balance and endurance.

Note: Home Workout
If you don't have a bench. A fitness ball is ok for flat press. Stay parallel to the ground and head always on the ball.

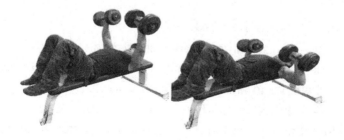

Flat Bench Chest Flies (dumbbells)

- Start with arms up over face, slightly bent elbows as if hugging a tree. Lock elbows with bend. Slowly lower dumbbells until your elbows are almost at bench height.
- Feet flat on floor or bent knees up and cross feet if a beginner. Squeeze pecks to bring weights back up and together (light touch). Squeeze Pecs on top (inside of pecs).
- Repeat. Only do after presses or main lifts.

Secondary Lift (Body Shaping Exercise).

Pros: builds inside of chest. Good for balance. Tip: place feet up, bent knee and cross ankles to work core, balance and chest.

Note: Home Workout
If you don't have a bench. A fitness ball is ok. Stay parallel to the ground and head always on the ball. Make sure that you perform flies so your elbows will touch the ball on the down position.

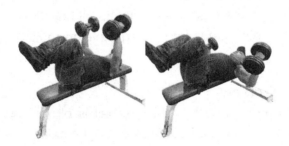

Overhead Pulls (dumbbells):

- This exercise targets upper chest and lats (sides of back if done correctly). Start with a dumbbell directly over your face. Pull elbows in and slightly bend elbows.
- Lock elbows in position. Squeeze upper chest and lower dumbbell behind head to get a good stretch in upper chest and lats. Make sure to emphasize elbows in.

- At bottom squeeze upper chest and lift dumbbell back to directly over face. Squeeze chest again. Repeat.

Pros: great exercise with heavier weight for upper chest after heavy lifts of flat bench (bar and/or dumbbell). Secondary exercise as is a body shaping lift.

Note: Home Workout
If you don't have a bench. A fitness ball is ok. Place upper back on ball and drop hips slightly. Your head must be on the ball.

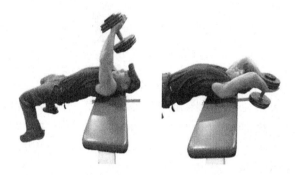

Incline Chest Press (dumbbells):

- Start with a bench at 45 degrees. Begin with weights at top over face. Slowly lower so your elbows are lowered to level of your shoulder.
- Squeeze upper peck and press dumbbells up with force. At top squeeze your chest as weights are on top, straight up. Don't bring weights together.

Primary Lift: build power, mass and balance.

Pro Tips: best done after flat bench bar or dumbbell. Emphasize upper chest. Follow up with a secondary exercise (incline flies), power push-ups, cable incline bench flies, decline push-ups, cable flies or lighter incline bar press for high reps.

Note: Home Workout

If you don't have a bench. A fitness ball is ok. Place back on ball and roll down so your hips are lower and your body is 45 degrees on the ball. Head should be on the ball.

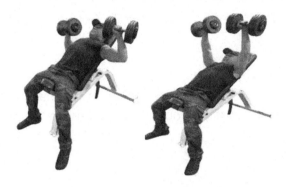

Incline Chest Flies (dumbbells):
- Start with a bench at 45 degrees. Begin with dumbbells parallel to each other over face. Lock out arms. Bend arms slightly as if wrapping arms around a cylinder. Lock elbows and arms into position.
- Lower dumbbells out and down to stretch pecs slowly. At end point, shoulder. Pause and bring dumbbells back to starting position.
- Emphasize the squeeze of your chest when on top.

Secondary Lift: body building and shaping, upper and inner chest.

Pro Tips: best done after heavy incline dumbbell or bar press. You can do small pulses on bottom to make strong contractions. Also, at the end of the exercise for the last few reps, as the dumbbells come together on top, turn the dumbbells inward so the ends touch to emphasize the inner chest.

Note: Home Workout
If you don't have a bench. A fitness ball is ok. Same as incline ball presses. Make sure head is on ball.

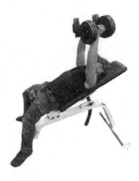

Dips:

- Start on a dip machine (body weight or gravitron: weight resistance dips. Begin with your body up over your hands, slightly leaning forwards with hips back to emphasize your chest not triceps.
- Bend arms so your elbows go straight back and your body goes down and forward to stretch your chest muscles.
- Contract your pecs and press to bring yourself back up (arms locked out on top). Down slow (negative) and explode up. Pause 1-2 seconds on top and repeat.

Primary Lift: top body weight exercise to build strength and pec density.

Pro-Tips: leaning forward focuses mostly chest and leaning back more vertical targets mostly triceps.

Best done after heavy bench day and/or as the main exercise in your body weight workout combined with pushups and arm exercises. Again, you can pulse on bottom or top to build muscle fibers. Also, you can add a dumbbell to the workout by crossing your ankles and holding the dumbbell in place between your ankles while you perform the exercise or use a dip chain to hold heavier weight for more resistance.

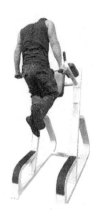 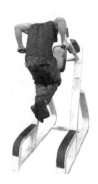

Flat Bench Press (Bar):

- Start with feet on solid surface (ground, plate or box) so you can press hard off heel. Back flat and hips down entire time. Hands slightly wider than shoulder width. Heels down at all times. Don't arch your back.
- Begin with bar over chest and arms locked out. Tight Grip on bar (this picture shows how bar is positioned on palm, make sure to make a fist).
- Let bar down slow and touch chest (between upper and lower) 1-2 seconds unless it's a pause routine (pause 3 seconds). Elbows can be slightly forward as you lower bar to take off pressure from shoulder with heavier weight. When pressing up make sure to dig your heels into the ground. Press heels harder when pressing bar up and back.
- As you press up make sure your elbows are directly under the bar. Press bar up and towards your face in arch movement. The key is to engage your upper back, triceps, and press off the heels as if pushing back.
- Once on top lock out elbows and wait 1-2 seconds before repeating.

Primary Lift: best for strength and bigger chest. Skip with any shoulder problem and exchange with dumbbells. Also, great for building tricep size and strength.

Pro-Tips: best done after warm up set with light weight. To build strength keeps reps low and weight heavier with a spotter. You can do pulses on the bottom at the end of a set to help grow your chest muscles. Also, perform pause pause sets on the days you perform high rep. Pause the bar on your chest 3 seconds then press up hard and fast. Weight should be 65-75% max.

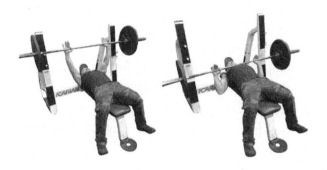

Incline Bench Press (Bar):

Start similar to the flat bench. Begin with back on a 45 degree angle. Use same method as for flat bench.

Primary Lift: same as flat.

PRO-TIPS: best done on same day as flat in different ratios. Heavy and low reps for flat. Lighter and higher reps for incline. Next workout, lighter and higher reps for flat and heavier and low reps for incline. To work upper chest you can do a few sets where bar almost hits top of your collar bone with lighter weight.

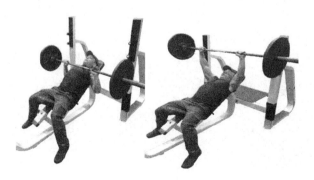

Push Ups

Push-Ups:

- Start with hands wide, fingers open and weight on palms of hands. Thumbs line up with shoulders. Feet wide, hip distance apart, to work abs. Variations: arms tucked in to sides works arms and shoulders. Keep abs tight entire time. Make sure not to arch back.
- Perform push-ups on knees if your form is not good while performing push-ups on your feet. Knees: keep knees in direct line with hips and shoulders.
- Perform a push-up as 1 unit.
- Inhale going down through your nose and exhale pressing up through your mouth.

PRO-TIPS: best push up is hands wider than shoulders and thumbs in-line with shoulders. You can perform push-ups every day. For muscle endurance, perform after heavy bench, in-between punching a heavy bag or after pull ups and dips.

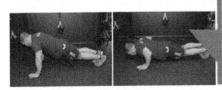

Power push ups: perform a push up and when on bottom position, spring off of ground with palms so your arms are straight, abs tight and palms raise 1-3 inches off ground. Land on palms and go down into bottom positon. Repeat.

Clapping push ups: are the best push up variation for arms, strength and endurance. Perform a power push up and clap before your palms touch ground.

Elevated Push Ups

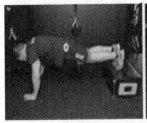
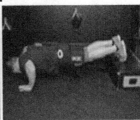
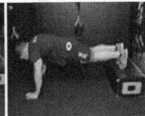

- Start same as push-ups. Place your balls of foot on a elevation 2- 12 inches. Increase height to increase resistance. Make sure lower back is straight.

Tricep Push Ups

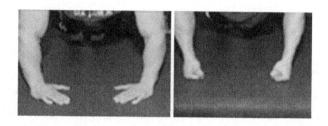

Start same as push-ups. Place your hands in triangle position. Hands should be directly under chest, neck or nose. Hands are best separated as seen above. Fingers at 45 degrees to prevent wrist injury. You can also work your triceps with a fist.

ARM EXERCISES

Tricep Rope Extensions:

- Start with feet together or hip distance apart. If feet together you'll keep elbows tight to side and stand up tall so you can bring handles straight up to your chest while keeping elbows pinned to your sides the entire time.
- Movement is from only your forearm going up and down. Key: lock out your elbow movement on bottom, pause 1-2 seconds and squeeze triceps. Go up slow and repeat.

Secondary Lift: best done after performing heavy bench or heavy tricep close grip press.

Variation 2: feet wider, lean over. Start with hands on chest and press them down and out away from each other like a reverse V. Lock out elbows on top and repeat.

Variation 3: one foot forward, lean over facing away from machine. Place handles together and behind your head. Press forward from behind head to over and in front of head with arms to full extension. Lock out elbows and squeeze triceps.

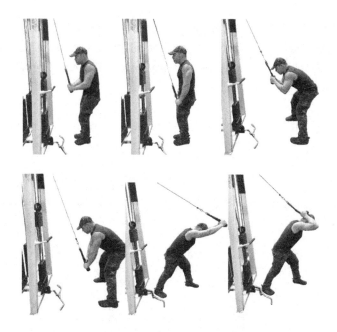

Pro-Tips: start with heavy reps and drop down in weight as you fatigue. At the end of the set finish with 10-20 small pulses where you squeeze triceps at full extension of arm. Example: 6 reps @ 100lb >10 reps @90lb>5-10 reps @80lb>10-20 small pulses. Make sure to squeeze triceps at end of lift. Follow up with power push-ups or clapping push-ups for endurance and strength.

If at home with no push down rope, you can perform kickbacks or dips.

DIPS: see chest exercises for description.

Overhead Tricep Extensions:

- Start with feet hip distance apart. Grab end of dumbbell with open palm and place your other palm over the other hand. Create an open cup with both hands to hold the dumbbell in vertical position overhead.
- Bend at the elbow so the dumbbell goes behind the head (try to keep dumbbell vertical) so the weight of the dumbbell is felt on the triceps. Make sure to keep your elbows tucked in and

back towards your head. Extend from the elbow by engaging your triceps. Once the dumbbell is overhead squeeze your triceps. Don't force the weight forward once overhead.

- Keep the dumbbell back.

Secondary Lift: perform after heavy bench, weighted dips or close grip triceps.

Pro-Tips: start with a heavier weight. Drop set with lighter weights after performing 6-8 reps @95% max. Follow up with more dips or power push-ups.

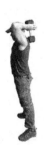 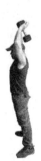

Tricep Close Grip Press:

- One of the best arm lifts for both strength and mass. Start by lying on a bench with feet hip distance apart and secure on floor. Set up same as if benching with a barbell. However, bring your hands inward so they are slightly narrower than shoulder distance apart.
- You'll initiate by bringing bar towards middle of chest and elbows down and back. All Tension should be on triceps and chest. Mostly triceps. If your shoulders or wrist hurt, place your hands out slightly wider.
- At full extension squeeze your triceps. Try not to bounce off chest once bar hits chest.

Primary Lift: mass and strength. This exercise will help build your bench press.

Pro-Tips: concentrate on this exercise if you want bigger arms and a stronger bench press. Perform mostly with heavier weights and less reps. Exceeding 15 reps may cause pain in your shoulder. Combine this with chest day. At the end of the exercise with a good spotter, perform pulses from your chest to 4-5 inches off chest and back down to chest for 3-5 reps then do a full rep and repeat 1-2 more times. Also, you can have a spotter help you lift it up but go down very slow resisting the downward motion (negative contraction). Once at chest have spotter help you lift up the weight.

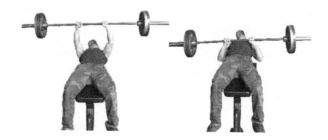

Tricep Bench Dips:

- Start with feet hip distance apart, hands on side of bench with palms on edge and fingers facing down. Hands should be next to hips. Back should be 1 inch from bench entire time.
- Start by bending at the elbow so your hips go below bench and press off your hands to extend your triceps fully on top of extension. You can place a heavy dumbbell on legs or place your feet up on an elevation to give yourself more resistance.
- Make sure your legs are slightly bent when placing your feet on an elevation.

Secondary Lift: this is similar to dips but not as effective to build mass. However, this is a great tricep exercise for home and to build arm endurance after performing heavy bench or heavy tricep close grip press.

Pro-Tips: use a heavy dumbbell on legs and perform 10-15 reps. Once fatigued, place the dumbbell down and perform as many as you can till failure or perform push-ups till failure.

Straight Bar Curls:

- Start with feet hip distance apart, hands on bar directly in front of shoulder, with back of hand on thighs. Your hands should not be next to hips.
- Start by contracting your bicep and bending at the elbow so elbows stay glued to your stomach. Palms should be directly in front of your shoulders at full range of motion.
- Contract bicep and hold squeeze 2 seconds. Let down at a slower rate 3-4 seconds causing an eccentric contraction (negative).

Primary Lift: this is a great mass building exercise for your arms. Best done heavy for at least 3-4 sets at low reps (4-8 reps) then lighter for more reps (10-12).

Pro-Tips: change it up with workouts. Perform low reps and heavy. Next workout perform heavy for low reps and drop set (lighten the weight) till you get to 20-30 reps. Also, once fatigued perform ½ reps and hold last rep at midpoint (static contraction, isometric for as long as you can). Also, another great set is to perform 6-8 heavy reps then follow with alternate dumbbell curls until fatigued at a lower rate for higher reps or time (1 minute).

** Note: can be done with a small bar on the cable machine. Best for burn out sets (perform reps to failure in drop set or pyramid set)

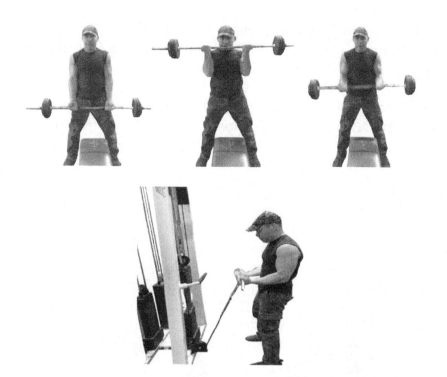

Standing REGULAR Dumbbell Curls (sitting or standing, standing is best for heavier weight but you won't isolate as much i.e. cheat):

- Similar to straight bar curls above. Start with feet hip distance apart, hands holding dumbbell, palm up, directly in front of shoulder, with back of hand on thighs OR dumbbell by your side if sitting. Start by contracting your bicep and bending at the elbow so elbows stay glued to your stomach or your side.
- Palms should be land directly in front of your shoulders whether you start with dumbbell on your thigh when standing or dumbbell is at your side when sitting.
- Contract bicep and hold squeeze 2 seconds. Let down at a slower rate 3-4 seconds causing an eccentric contraction (negative).

Primary Lift: this is a great mass building exercise for your arms. Best done heavy for at least 3-4 sets at low reps (4-8 reps) then lighter for more reps (10-12).

Pro-Tips: Don't turn dumbbells up at top. Keep the tension on bicep entire time. Change it up by performing a regular curl (palm up) then a hammer curl (vertical) and repeat. Also, pulses work well at end of set when fatigued (pulse full to half or stay at half and go a little down and back to half for 5-15 reps). Another good way to build bicep muscle endurance is to perform chin ups immediately after performing bicep curls.

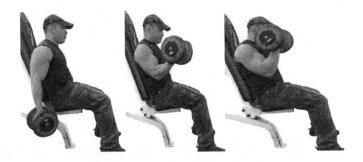

Standing HAMMER Curls (sitting or standing, standing is best for heavier weight but you won't isolate as much i.e. cheat):

- Start with feet together when standing, palms facing thighs and dumbbell grip vertical. Your hands should be next to hips. Elbows and arms locked to your sides to start.
- Start by contracting your bicep and bending at the elbow. Once your hands go ½ way up your elbows will rise up and forward but make sure to keep them pinned to your ribs as much as possible.
- Dumbbell head should tap front of shoulder. Contract bicep and hold squeeze 2 seconds. Let down at a slower rate 3-4 seconds causing an eccentric contraction (negative).

Primary Lift: this is a great mass building exercise for your arms. Best done heavy for at least 3-4 sets at low reps (4-8 reps) then lighter for more reps (10-12).

Pro-Tips: best alternative to straight bar or regular curls if you have a wrist injury. Perform sets and reps similar to regular curl. Perform after straight bar. You can also perform this with a rope on the cable machine at the gym for drop sets or high reps and low weight (30-50 reps) when doing a burn out set at the end of a workout or to increase muscular endurance.

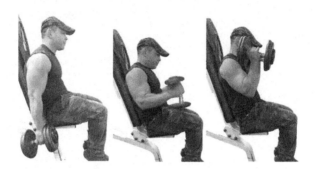

Concentration Curls:

- Sit on a bench. Place opposite hand on thigh. Place your elbow on top of your hand so it fits in the corner created with your hand on the thigh for support.
- Keep the palm of your hand in position to be angled towards your shoulder from extension to full contraction. Isolate the bicep. Best done with heavier weight then dropping down to lighter weight.
- Contract bicep exercise at top and hold 2 sec as if posing. Let down slowly with resistance.

Secondary Lift: this is a great isolation exercise for shaping your bicep. Best done after heavy straight bar or heavy regular dumbbell curls.

Pro-Tips: drop set and pulses toward the end of failure. Go back and forth from arm to arm for all sets before moving on to next exercise. You can use your other hand or spotter to do that last rep.

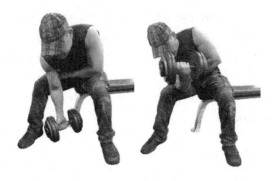

BACK EXERCISES

Close Grip Pulls:

- Sit with knees locked in. Place hands shoulder width apart, palms facing you with full grip. Squeeze lats (side of back) to initiate pulling from fully extended straight arm over head to pulling bar under chin right to sternum under chin.
- Once on chest squeeze lats 2-3 seconds then release to bring hands back to starting position overhead.
- Make sure you'll pull bar down hard and fast and release up slow 3-4 seconds (negative contraction). Also, weight should always be heavy and challenging

Secondary Lift: this is a great isolation exercise for shaping your lats but can be a primary exercise if you lift heavy for 6-8 reps to put on mass for the lats. Best done after heavy one arm row, low-row or deadlift.

Pro-Tips: use heavy weight and perform 6-8 reps then go lighter and do another 10 reps. Last rep hold and pulse bar 4-5 inches from chest and back to chest till failure. **Also, another great tip** is to let elbows flair out when bar is going up and tuck them in when pulling down. Follow up with chin ups for endurance or weighted chin ups for mass.

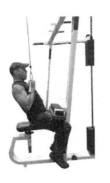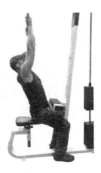

Wide Grip Pulls:

- Sit with knees locked in. Place hands wider than shoulder width apart, palms facing away with full grip. IMPORTANT: try to stay locked into position (45 degrees or straight up when pulling down, although you can cheat with very hard weight to get a few more reps in by leaning back while pulling bar down).
- Squeeze lats (side of back) to initiate pulling from fully extended straight arm over head to pulling bar under chin right to upper chest and/or under chin. Once on chest squeeze lats 2-3 seconds then release to bring hands back to starting position overhead.
- Make sure you'll pull bar down hard and fast and release up slow 3-4 seconds (negative contraction). Also, weight should always be heavy and challenging.

Secondary Lift: this is a great isolation exercise for shaping your lats and upper back but can be a primary exercise if you lift heavy for 6-8 reps to put on mass for the lats. Best done after heavy one arm row, low row or deadlift. Follow up

Pro-Tips: use heavy weight and perform 6-8 reps then go lighter and do another 10 reps. Last rep hold and pulse bar 4-5 inches from chest and back to chest till failure. **Also, another great tip** is to combine this with heavy low rows. Perform heavy low row and run over to this exercise for more reps and lighter weight.

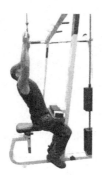
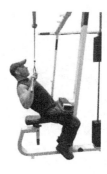

One Arm Row:

- Start with one knee on bench and the other foot wider than hip distance to side of bench, knee slightly bent. Palm on bench to support should be placed so fingers go over edge. Lean forward over supporting harm. Hold dumbbell and let arm hang.
- Pull dumbbell straight up and hold on top 2-3 seconds. Alternate Stance: 3-point stance square to support and feet hip distance apart, see pic.
- Squeeze lats before pulling up, hold up on top 2-3 seconds. Let dumbbell down slow and pull up with intensity.

Primary Lift: this is a primary exercise to put on mass for the lats and upper back. Best done with heavy low row and/or deadlift.

Pro-Tips: use heavy weight and perform 6-8 reps then go lighter and do another 10 reps. Also, a great set is perform 5 each arm and repeat for another 4-5 sets without resting. For a burner, perform bent over raises and/or wide grip or v-bar pull ups.

Regular Stance

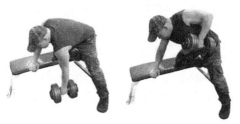

3-Point Stance

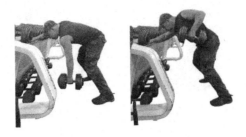

Low Row:

- Start by sitting on bench, slightly bent legs, grab v-bar or straight bar directly in front of you with straight arms.
- Engage lats, upper back and pull bar to your chest (upper or middle). Squeeze upper back and lats once bar is at chest. Hold 2-3 seconds and then release slowly till arms are out in front. Repeat.

Primary Lift: this is a primary exercise to put on mass for the lats and upper back. Combine with one arm row and dead lifts to add mass.

Pro-Tips: lift heavy. Follow-up with lighter weight and/or pull ups. Change it up with the bar, drop sets, pyramiding, pulsing and varying reps.

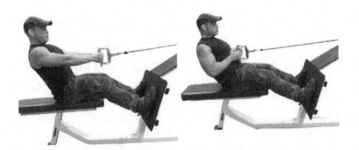

Power Pull Ups:

- Chin Up (palms facing you, shoulder width) or Pull Ups (palms facing away, 2-3 inches wider than shoulder width).

Stand under bar with feet on ground or on a box. You should be able to jump off the box and explode up as you pull up.

- Drop straight down with straight legs. Don't let your body swing. Explode off the platform and pull up once your feet hit the ground. This is like a plyometric exercise.
- Make sure you use your upper body for the exercise. The legs are too assist to perform for the entire time in program i.e. 30 sec or 1 min.

Primary Lift: Great for increasing upper body strength.

Pro-Tips: great for traveling and to increase upper body endurance if done after a weight exercise like straight bar curls, close grip pulls, etc..

SHOULDER EXERCISES

Bent Over Raises:

- Start by sitting on edge of bench. Bend forward, let dumbbells hang below legs. Back should be almost 45 degrees. Dumbbells can be horizontal or vertical (see pics below).
- Engage upper back and squeeze scapula to raises dumbbells up and back. Weight should be light enough that you can hold lift 1-2 seconds at top. Let Down slow.

Secondary Lift: isolation exercise. Great for increasing mass but also creating cuts between shoulder blades and back of shoulder.

Pro-Tips: you can lift heavier for a few set by cheating, lift and let go down. Drop weight to then perform with great form. Follow low-row with bent over raises to isolate the upper back.

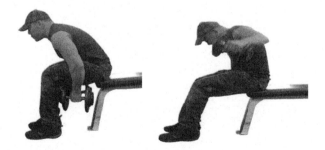

Horizontal Position

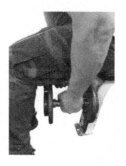

Vertical Position (allows more depth between scapula)

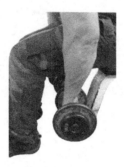

Shoulder Press (dumbbells):

- Start standing or sitting with feet hip distance apart and arms 90 degrees to ground. Press dumbbells straight up to lock out elbows to full extension above head.
- Drive up with power and fast but controlled. Let down slow. Don't let elbows drop more than 1 inch below shoulder and don't bring weights together above head as this may pinch nerve in neck with heavier weights and also lets off tension on shoulder.

Primary Lift: great for building mass and bowling ball shoulders.

Pro-Tips: best done after straight bar shoulder press with bar. This really activates your shoulder muscle fibers. Also, perform this exercise with lighter weights and more reps to build muscular endurance. Vary with drop sets (heavy to light) and pyramid sets (light to heavy).

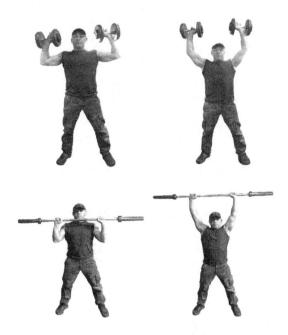

Upright Rows (dumbbells and bar):

- Start standing with feet hip distance apart. Grab bar or dumbbells with hands3-5 inches apart and palms facing in (see pics). If your wrist bothers you, hold dumbbells or bar slightly wider grip.
- Pull dumbbells or bar 1-2 inches from under chin, hold 2-3 seconds and let down slower 2-3 seconds (negative contraction). Make sure to explode up with a heavier weight.
- This exercise is best done with heavier weight and low reps. Builds your traps and delts.
- Explosive Upright Row: squat slightly forward, hang dumbbells and explode up with legs and pulling up dumbbells at same time similar to a power clean.

Primary Lift: great for building mass for shoulders and traps.

Pro-Tips: best done with straight bar than follow up with dumbbells. Also, I like to have clients alternate this exercise with heavy shrugs for 10-15 reps (drop set for both shrugs and upright rows). For a more explosive upright row, add your legs to the movement (see pic).

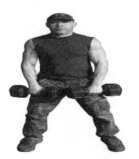 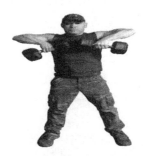

Explosive Upright Row:

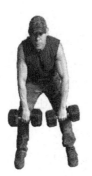 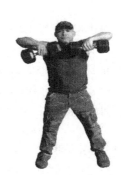

Shrugs (dumbbell or bar):
- Hold dumbbells with straight, locked arms by your side (palms facing legs). Keeping arms straight entire time, shrug shoulders up towards ears with explosive power and hold on top 2-3 seconds squeezing traps, let down slow and repeat.
- Bar: hold bar with overhand grip (palms facing your legs) shoulder width apart.
- Shrug shoulders up to ear, straight arms and locked elbows, hold 2-3 seconds on top squeezing traps, let down slow and repeat.

Primary Lift: best for traps with heavier weight. Follow up with upright row to get a good pump for neck.

Pro-Tip: alternate exercises or even every other rep between shrugs and upright row. Example: shrug for a rep then upright row for a rep and repeat.

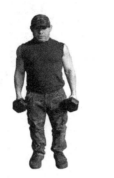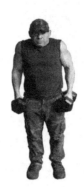

Shoulder Side Raises (dumbbells):

- Start standing or sitting with feet hip distance apart and arms by your side. Raise dumbbells from hip to shoulder height.
- Once at shoulder height. Hold for 2 seconds than lower slowly till touches lightly on leg.

Secondary Lift: great for shaping your side delts.

Pro-Tips: best done in combination with front shoulder raises. You can start with arms 90 degrees and dumbbells in front of you to raise your elbows up and out. This will allow you to use heavier weight and add more mass to your side delts.

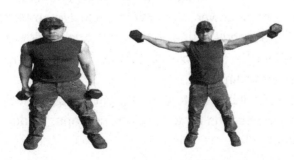

Shoulder Front Raises (dumbbells or plate):

- Start standing with feet hip distance apart and arms in front with dumbbells resting on thigh. Raise dumbbells from thigh to shoulder height. Once at shoulder height.
- Hold for 2 seconds than lower slowly till touches lightly on leg.

Secondary Lift: great for shaping your front delts.

Pro-Tips: great in combination with side shoulder raises. Also, best when done after heavy shoulder press with either bar or dumbbells for a burn out set. Perform shoulder front raises along with dumbbell raises in the same workout. Keep arms 90% straight and locked. Raise above your head and back down slowly.

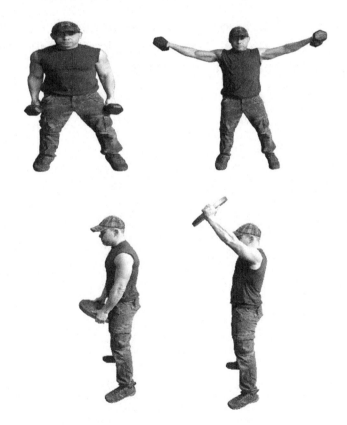

Plate Front Raises (guy # 2 especially)

Squat and Press (dumbbells):

- Start standing with feet hip distance apart and dumbbells resting vertical on shoulders next to ears, elbows tucked in. Squat on heels and press dumbbells straight up while you stand.
- Lock out arms over head.

Important: bring dumbbells back down to shoulders in starting position BEFORE squatting.

Primary Lift: great for building strength and size as this allows you to lift heavier dumbbells as you are using your entire body to press weights overhead.

Pro-Tips: best done for low reps and heavy weights 90% max 4-5 reps. Once done with set, immediately perform 6-10 more reps of either dumbbell or bar press overhead @ 70-80% max.

LEG EXERCISES

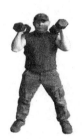 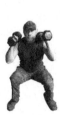 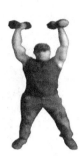

Back Squats (bar):

- Start standing with feet slightly wider than hip distance apart and toes turned slightly out. Bar resting above scapula, not on C7 vertebrae (bony protrusion in upper back) or neck.
- Breathe in through nose keeping abs engaged and breadth in to help stabilize lower abs and back. Squat pressing back on heels while leaning slightly forward so you land in 45 degree angle with a straight back, not rounded.
- Make sure to go down slower and not bounce off the bottom. Eyes forward and head slightly back. Once your butt goes below parallel or parallel, press off heals and power up.
- Stand on top and lockout hips. Wait 2 seconds and repeat.

Primary Lift: best leg exercise for endurance with higher reps and mass with low to high reps. Strength builder for entire lower body and biochemically for upper body too.

Pro-Tips: best done in combination with leg press at the gym or jumping squat at home. Drop setting or pyramid sets are great to build endurance and mass. Make sure to wear a narrow belt if lifting heavy. Best to progress slowly week by week with heavier weight. If your shoulder hurts or you have lower back issues, then use a dumbbell. Smith Machine squats: you'll perform same but your feet should be slightly forward in front of you and parallel instead of slightly turned out. Great to do heavy bar squats then immediately follow up with smith machine squats for higher reps.

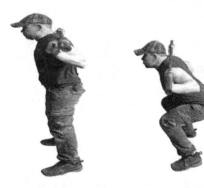

Front Step Ups (dumbbells):

- Start with one foot (make sure entire foot is on bench) and other on ground. Your knee should be aligned 90 degrees to hip when foot is on bench (foot on bench and knee 90 degrees from hip to knee). If not, then place a mat or something to bring foot higher from ground.
- To initiate exercise, press off heel on bench and lock out leg that's up on bench completely before stepping up from floor to bench. Once completely standing erect on bench with both feet. Step down with same foot that was on ground and repeat for reps in program.
- When finished with that leg, switch to other leg. Hold dumbbells by your side entire time with locked out arms so legs do entire exercise.

Secondary Lift: great for home workouts to build quads after lifting heavy squats. Example: 10 bar squats @85% max followed by 15 step ups holding dumbbells @ 80% max.

Pro-Tips: perform for low reps 8-12 or 15-25 each leg dependent on goal. Higher reps are great for sport oriented programs. Perform in combination with side step ups (see below).

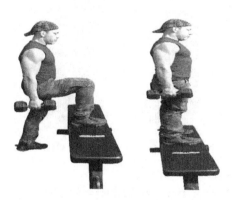

Side Step Ups (dumbbells):

- Similar to front step ups. Start with one foot (make sure entire foot is on bench) and other on ground. Your knee should be aligned 90 degrees to hip when foot is on bench (foot on bench and knee 90 degrees from hip to knee). If not, then place a mat or something to bring foot higher from ground.
- To initiate exercise, press off heel on bench and lock out leg that's up on bench completely before stepping up from floor to bench. Once completely standing erect on bench with both feet. Step down with same foot that was on ground and repeat for reps in program.
- When finished with that leg, switch to other leg. Hold dumbbells by your side entire time with locked out arms so legs do entire exercise.

Secondary Lift: great for home workouts to build quads after lifting heavy squats. Example: 10 bar squats @85% max followed by 15 step ups holding dumbbells @ 80% max. Then perform the front step us with the same reps and weight.

Pro-Tips: perform for low reps 8-12 or 15-25 each leg dependent on goal. Higher reps are great for sport oriented programs.

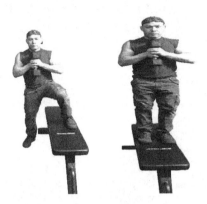

Alternating Lunges (dumbbells):

- Start with feet hip distance apart, not together. Hold dumbbells by your side with straight arms. Step out and forward with right leg onto the right heel (make sure you step out far enough so the back knee drops down to 1 inch off the ground and the front knee is 90 degrees from your shit to the thigh.
- The front knee should stay behind the front toe if you drop a straight line down from knee to toes. If not, lean back more or step out a little further. Make sure hips are under your legs and you're not leaning forward.
- Drive off the heel NOT the toes in the front foot to go back to standing position. Repeat with other leg.

Secondary Lift: great for home workouts to build quads after lifting heavy squats and building endurance in legs.

Pro-Tips: pyramid from heavy to low dumbbells and stay at 5 -10 reps each leg. Then drop down in weight 2-3 more times with lighter weights for 5-10 reps each time. Also, you can walk and lunge which is similar but do for time or long distance. Make sure to keep feet hip distance apart and step straight out not at an angle.

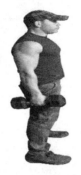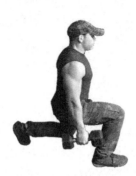

Stand Ups (dumbbells):

- Start with both knees on a mat. Hold a dumbbell horizontal under chin. Start by stepping up with right foot in front of you as if in a lunge.
- Press off your right heel to stand up straight. Now, kneel back down with the right knee and then the left knee. Repeat all on the right side for reps in the program.
- Now perform the left leg for the same reps. Don't step out to the side and make sure to step out far enough so all weight presses off your front heel that you stepped out.

Secondary Lift: great for home workouts to build quads after lifting heavy squats.

Pro-Tips: perform with or in exchange of squats if you don't have access to heavy weight for squats. Perform 10-25 each leg holding 10-30lb dumbbell and perform jumping squats with a weight 10-15 reps and then jog 1 mile and repeat 2-4x.

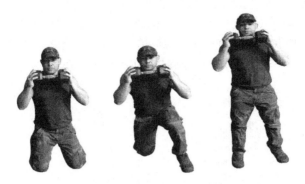

Goblet, Front Squat (dumbbells):

- Start with both feet hip distance apart with feet slightly turned out. Squat so your weight goes back over heels, not toes, and your shoulders lean forward.
- Squat until your bum goes 1 inch below knee level and your elbows touch knees. Press off your heels to rise straight up. At top, lock out your hips by pushing hips forward. Repeat.

Primary Lift: great for home workouts to build legs without much equipment. Bar squats are superior but heavy dumbbell squats are effective for building both endurance and strength.

Pro-Tips: perform 6-10 reps @ 90% max and follow immediately with one of the following exercises at home: jump rope (running), lunges, weighted jump and squat, sprints or jumping jacks.

Leg Press:

- Start with back support at lowest level, usually 45 degrees. Lower back always supported and against the back support. NEVER roll it up off the platform as your bringing down the platform to press back up.
- Feet can be different positions to work different parts of your legs. Parallel and straight to train your quads and strength. Feet wide and turned out to target inner thighs. Toes out and heels together with feet higher up on platform to target hamstrings and quads.

- In-hale while bringing weight down and breathe out as pressing weight up. Pause on top and repeat.

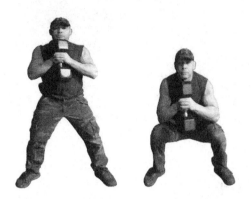

Primary Lift: mostly a gym exercises due to the leg press machine. Great for pressing heavy weights after squats. Combine heavy sets of 4-6 reps with endurance sets of 12-25 reps.

Pro-Tips: perform most of your sets with feet parallel. Combine with heavy squat sets. After 6-10 heavy reps you can bring to bottom and pulse ½ way to the top and back down to bottom position or pulse ½ way to the top position. Calf Raises: leg press can be used as in picture for calf raises.

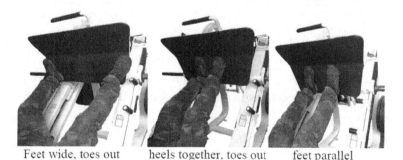

Feet wide, toes out   heels together, toes out   feet parallel

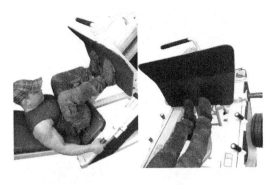

Bottom position   calf raises

Back Leg Curl:

- Start lying flat on stomach, hold bars below pad. Make sure your knees hang 1 inch over edge of pad. Pad should be on your Achilles (behind heel) and toes pull up towards you (flexed at all times). Engage glutes and hamstrings to pull heels up to butt, hold 2 seconds and let down slow 2-4 seconds.

- Once at bottom power back up and repeat. Perform with good form and make sure not to use heavier weight than you can perform less than 6 reps (prone to tendon pull if done too heavy or poor form).

Secondary Lift: mostly a gym exercise due to the back leg machine. Great for targeting hamstrings and shaping hamstrings. Use in conjunction with heavy squats, deadlifts and good mornings. Pyramid the weight from heavy to light for best results. Always perform a warm up set (light and high reps) and stretch hamstrings well before starting with heavier weights.

Pro-Tips: make sure feet are parallel. To target high up on hamstrings you can curl toes up as your pulling bar up towards your butt and flex feet down as your lowering bar. Make sure to use lighter weight and low reps if you decide to do this targeting tip. At end of heavy set you can pulse the bar from butt to 6 inches and back up to butt for another 8-12 reps.

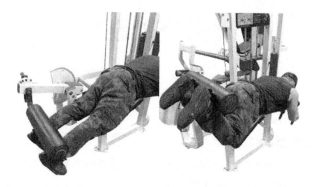

AB EXERCISES

Plank On Ball:

- Place forearms on a 55 to 65 cm fitness ball. Keep chest and belly off of ball at all times.
- Feet shoulder width (increases core engagement and balance)
- Hold for 1-5 minutes as in your program.

Ball Roll Out:

- Same position as plank on the ball. The difference is you're rolling your forearms and elbows away from starting position and back to start 1-3 inches.
- Make sure not to roll beyond 3-4 inches as this may cause a lower back injury. Keep feet wide and stabilize your lower back.

Secondary Ab Exercises: this is a great exercise to perform after regular sit ups to engage your lower abs and core.

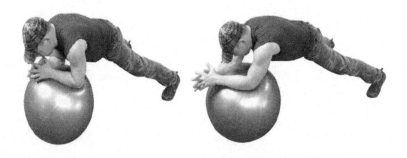

Kick Outs:

- Place feet in table top position (bend knees, feet held up knee height, toes pointed). Flex up hard (crunch) **and stay flexed!**
- Engaging abs the entire time, inhale and kick legs out hard at 45 degrees. Inhale and draw knees in.
- Repeat in and out for the time and/or reps in program.

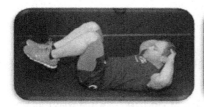 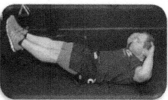

45 Degree Crunches:

- Place feet in table top position (bend knees, feet held up knee height, toes pointed). Flex up hard (crunch) **and stay flexed!**
- Engaging abs the and keeping your legs up at 45 degrees the entire time. Perform small crunches until your abs or lower back get tired.
- Once you can't perform anymore. Start over. This exercises is very challenging so you should feel it within 15 to 30 seconds. Repeat crunching for the time and/or reps in program.

Ball Crunches:

- Lie on the ball with lower back supported. Start with upper body in table top position (parallel to floor).
- Hands on ears. Important: engage abs and then crunch straight up and forward. Crunches should be small and tight like pulsing.
- Keep hips up by pressing off the floor with your heels.
- Notice how the movement comes from flexing abs while pressing back into the ball.

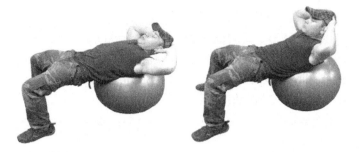

Hops:

- Lying flat with legs straight up towards ceiling with toes pulled toward you (flexed). Legs straight as possible.
- Hands by your side, palms flat on the ground next to your hip.
- Head down, engage abs, push slightly off the ground press hips off the ground towards ceiling. Press heels, not toes, up. Don't rock back.
- Keep hips up by pressing off the floor with your heels (heels should be flat when pressing up as if placing foot on ceiling).
- Hold up 2 seconds and let down slow. Repeat.

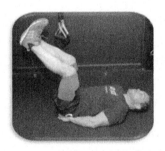 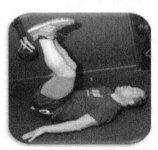

Sit Ups:

- First, sit ups work great if done correctly. However, if you have a lower back problem, then you must be careful. Also, if you have tight hip flexors I recommend scooting back so theres more distance between your butt and your heels.
- Always, start in a crunch position so your chin is 1 inch from your chest, hands on ears and abs engaged. You should be

looking over your knees. Hands on ears entire time with elbows slightly wide.

- Engage abs and sit up until you are almost vertical. Never look down. At top slowly roll down one vertebrae at a time.
- Most important, land in a crunch position and immediately repeat your sit up.
- DON'T! let your hand fall back and disengage abs by coming out of your crunch. Don't let head snap back. You should never be looking at the ceiling when you are in the starting position.

Sit Up Options:

- Sit ups with a medicine ball on your chest.
- Sit up with a twist (hands on ears) twist opposite elbow to opposite knee. Don't bend down to touch elbow to the knee. Sit up tall and cross over knee with elbow.
- Sit ups with punch, punch. Same as twist but you'll punch up and over the opposite knee. Twist and punch, bring back the hand to cheek and twist to the other side and punch. Go back to neutral and roll back down.

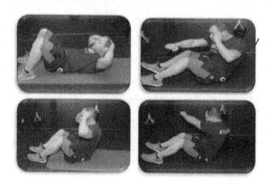

Leg Flutter:

- Start flexed up or head down on ground. Hands under butt for support, knees bent in table top position with feet pointed.

- Kick your pointed toes and legs straight out 45 degrees till locked out.
- Start to flutter one foot up and one down for amount of time in program.

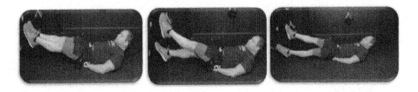

Optional:

Leg Lifts: bring both feet up and down at the same time from 90 degrees to the floor with feet flexed (toes pulled towards you). Lower slowly, tap the floor lightly and bring up fast.

Bicycle:
- Start flexed up, knees bent, hands on ears, elbows out wide and engage abs before starting with a crunch.
- Initiate by kicking one leg out, pointed toe, and other legs gets pulled in. Simultaneously, rotate opposite shoulder to the opposite leg and imagine touching your elbow to the opposite knee.
- You should have abs engaged and flexed so you can't physically touch knee to opposite elbow.
- Kick legs out and knees scrape together as one foot kicks out (pointed toe) to 45 degrees and other drives towards your chest. Repeat back and forth.

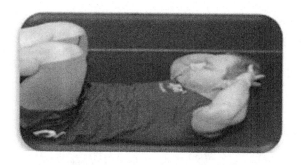

Flexed Position Before Starting the Bicycle.

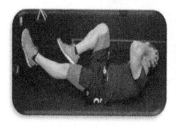 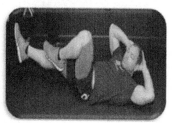

Hanging Leg Raises:

- Hold yourself up in a vertical position with your arms on the arm pads, straps or holding onto pull up bar.
- Drive knees straight up to chest or chin level.
- Hold 2-3 seconds and lower your legs slowly.

Options:

- Explosive Raises: with straps: place box under your feet or if skip the box if your feet can touch the ground. Drive off the box or ground hard to drive knees up hard and fast. Repeat for 30 seconds to 1 minute without rest. Make sure your feet hit box or ground directly in front of your and not behind you.
- Straight Leg Raises: Don't bend the knees and lift your legs up and out till your feet are in front and your legs are 90 degrees you're your upper body.
- Side Bend: Keep knees together and raises knees and feet up towards your right and also towards your left to focus on your obliques (sides).

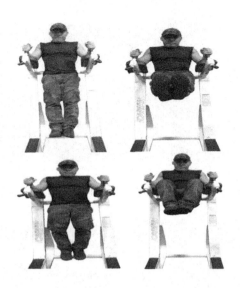

CARDIO

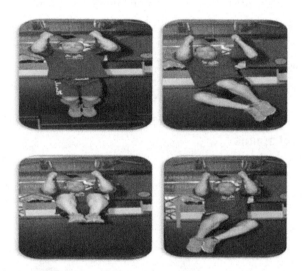

Rope (use a heavy rope if possible, 40 plus pounds):

Alternate Swing: start by holding on each end. Squat down and hold the squat. Lean slightly forward and raise the right hand while dropping the left. Stay loose with your arms and snap the rope up and down as fast as possible.

Primary Cardio: this is a must have for home or the gym to build muscle endurance. Always buy a quality and heavy rope. Most gyms have a very light rope (20-30 pound) which will not work as well.

Pro-Tips: make sure to whip arms up and down. Keep core engaged, breathe and stay in a squat position. You can add a squat up and down to work legs while simultaneously chopping rope up and down.

Rope Slam:

- Start by holding the rope on each end. Bring arms up over head with straight arms and slam both rope ends down at same time. Make sure to slam it hard.
- Best To stand and while slamming the rope simultaneously squat and drop your body. Everything drops.
- Make sure to keep arms overhead then slam with arms straight but not locked out.

Pro-Tips: use a heavier rope and use your technique and just not muscle. Great to add to shoulder or arm day. Also, perform after push-ups and sprints.

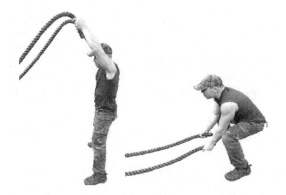

Rope Slams: Bring your arms over head and notice how I squat at the same time as slamming the rope hard using my triceps and shoulders. Drop down. Don't bend over to slam the rope. Don't pull the rope back. Keep the rope lose so the rope is not taught.

Alternate Rope Chop

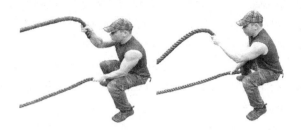

Star Jumps:

- Tuck down to a forward, low squat as if downhill skiing with arms pulled in, feet together and hands under chin.
- Jump up (explode) up high while pressing arms overhead in a Y shape and legs spread out far and away from your center. Bring your arms and legs back into starting position before landing.
- Touch ground in front as your starting position to make it more difficult.

Primary Cardio: this can replace all burpees. Burpees overall can be harmful to your lower back.

Pro-Tips: perform after heavy squats, lunges or leg press to build your endurance. Replace burpees with star jumps especially if you have a shoulder or lower back injury.

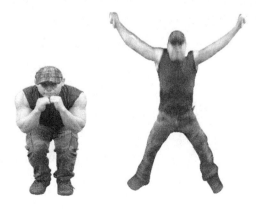

Kettle Bell Swing:

- Start by squatting and grabbing the kettle bell directly under you with both hands. Lift and hinge forward. The motion should come from your hips exploding forward and back.
- You should use very little arm or shoulder strength. The exercise is all from a pendulum type of motion. Get a rhythm with your breath.
- Keep your core engaged the entire time and work on speed along with a consistent tempo.
- Swing the kettle bell or Vertical Dumbbell through the legs with press back of your hips and swing the kettle bell above eye level with a swing of the hips forward.

Primary Cardio: this is a must have for home or the gym. You should buy 1-3 kettle bells that vary from 15-30 pounds. Thus, you can vary it up with one hand, 2 hands, hang and clean and power lifts, just to name a few.

Pro-Tips: speed and mobility are more important than just poundage to get the benefits of a kettle bell swing. You should work on great form before moving up in weight. A 15 pound kettle bell is fine for starting with a basic kettle bell 2-handed swing for 1-2 minutes. The kettle bell in the picture happens to be 60lbs.

NOTE: you can hold a dumbbell in a vertical position if you don't have a kettle bell. Hold the handle with one hand over the other. Don't hold the end of the dumbbell.

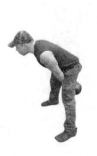 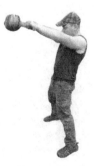

Back N' Forth:

- Start with both feet on one side of either a cone, line or rope. Feet can be together or separate (best for previous knee injuries).
- You'll crouch 1-2 inches down and stay in that position while you jump right to left over the object as fast as you can.
- Keep hands up entire time.

Primary Cardio: this is an easy way to increase coordination and stamina anywhere.

Pro-Tips: best to add to a cardio circuit. Also, perform after heavy squats, lunges or leg press to increase muscle endurance.

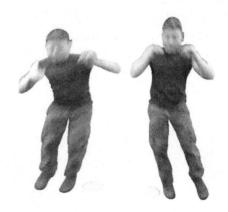

Bosu X-Overs:

- Start by placing your right foot on the Bosu and the left foot on the ground. Now, pick up your right foot and stamp it down on the Bosu to push up in the air by extending your right leg straight and simultaneously pressing off the ground with your left foot to go up and hop over.
- You'll now do the same with your left foot on the Bosu and repeat to go back and forth. Keep your hands up on your chin and elbows tucked into your sides the entire time.

Primary Cardio: this is one of the best exercises to build leg stamina especially for fighters. Perform this between rounds of punching or immediately after sprinting for 1-5 minutes without rest.

Pro-Tips: make sure to think about springing up more than going right to left fast. Explode up.

NOTE: you can also use a box 12-14 inches and do the same. Not as effective but can work in exchange of the Bosu.

No Bosu on hand? Then replace with a skate. Place both feet together. Squat and lean forward. Stay squatted and lean forward the entire time. Press off your right foot to spring over to the left and once you hit the ground spring back right by pressing of the left foot. Make sure to press off the heel and side of your foot, not the toes. You should feel your lateral leg from pushing. Lean forward so your shoulders are over your toes. All The weight should be on your legs and butt.

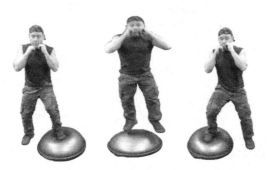

Power Skip: start skipping with intensity. Explode up as high as possible with one leg. Focus on the up rather than forward movement. Reach with the opposite hand while skipping up.

Primary Cardio: this is a great exercise to increase leg stamina and leg power.

Pro-Tips: perform power skips in the same workout as sprinting, bounding and squats.

NOTE: If you don't have the time to make it to the field or open area. Perform a basketball layup with 2 steps, turn and repeat as stated in program.

Bounding:

- Start in a squat position, arms straight behind you, hands in knife hand position (palms facing each other behind you). Throw arms straight up and forward in front of you to spring (explode forward) up and out off of toes in a leaping manner.
- Land as far as possible by leaping forward using your leg strength. Land softly into a squat. Stand up, wait 2 seconds and start over. Start over as if performing each one as it's the first.
- Concentrate on giving it your all for each one.

Primary Cardio: this is a great explosive plyometric that will build both stamina and leg power. Perform on a field or give yourself 10 to 15 feet of

open space. After performing each one, turn and repeat back and forth.

Pro-Tips: make sure to think about springing up and forward. Explode from a squat position by using leg power and forward positioning of arm swing. Make sure to rest 2-3 seconds before repeating another bound. Suggestion: bound with a weighted medicine ball 20-50 yards. Also, bound 25-30 yards and sprint back to starting position.

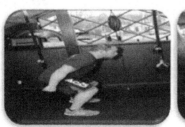 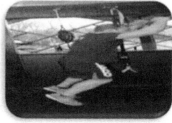

Sprinting:

- Sprinting is a superior cardio exercise for muscle endurance, power (leg and upper body) and to build cardio capacity (Oxygen exchange at the cellular level). However, you must progress slowly. Don't sprint at 100% power within the first 1 to 2 weeks of developing your sprinting program.
- Always warm up with a slow jog, 10-15 minutes of stretching (especially calves, hamstring, quads, lower and upper back). Power off your legs and utilize upper body by swinging your arms in a pendulum movement opposite of the opposing leg.
- Driving off with a forward position and keeping chest up high. Focus on driving elbows back and forward and hold fingers together as if holding a thing piece of paper between your index finger and thumb.
- Keep your upper body light and fluid. All the focus is driving off your glutes, hamstring, calves and quads

Burpees (Down Ups):

- Start with feet hip distance apart. Drop down on the balls of your feet and place your hands next to feet.
- Palms down. Kick your legs back hip distance apart. Keep your abs tight and straighten your legs.
- Don't arch back. Drop your entire body down to the ground and press off your palms hard to spring up in order to pop your feet back under your hips into a squat position.
- Stand up tall and repeat or jump straight up into the air.

NOTE: you can perform a push up rather than dropping your body to the ground.

IMPORTANT: NEVER perform burpees with either a past or present knee or lower back injury. Burpees can cause back injury. Perform burpees slowly and take your time. Focus on the push off the ground with your upper body to spring up onto your feet not toes.

Lower Back Issue? Exchange burpees with star jumps. I personally Recommend star jumps over burpees because they are very effective and cause far less injury.

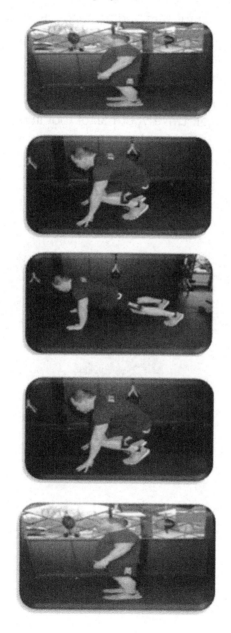

Mountain Climbers:

- Start on hands, chest up, drop hips and place pressure on palms of hands at all times.
- Place one foot forward and one back. Knees pulled in so you drive knees up to chest (scrape knees together as one goes up and other back). Don't bounce hips up and down while driving feet up and back.
- Make sure you fornt foot hits the ground at the same time as your back foot. Drive your ball of foot into the ground at the same time. Don't dangle the front foot in the air. Remember, you're driving up a mountain.
- Don't tap the ground lightly. Keep hips down. Your back knee should be about 1-2 inches from the ground Make sure your ball of feet are both into the ground, not in the air!

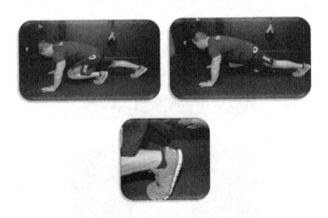

BOXING

Stance: basic stance with your lead foot forward and your strong hand back. Either an orthodox or South Paw foot body position.

Orthodox Stance: the majority of boxers will be an Orthodox stance with their left hand forward (lead hand) and their right hand back (power hand).

South Paw Stance: your right hand forward (lead hand) and your Left hand back (power hand.

How to Set Up Your Stance:
1. Start with feet hip distance apart. Step back with your strong hand foot. Stand on the balls of your feet, not tippy toes.
2. Turn both feet 45 degrees and go on to the balls of your feet, not toes. Lift your heels but keep your weight back on them. You should feel like you could sprint at any time. Your back foot should NEVER be perpendicular to your body.
3. Keep equal weight on both legs and your legs under your hips unless throwing hooks to the body.
4. Bring hands up at eye level and keep elbows in. Your body needs to be loose when punching. Don't muscle your punches.
5. Fist closed tight when punching.
6. Lead hip and lead shoulder facing your opponent.
7. Don't square up

Power Tips:

- Train in both stance. Become a skilled fighter by throwing punches from both sides. Best to stay in your strongest stance.
- Try to train with hands up always.

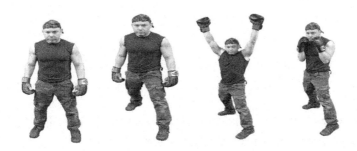

How to Jab:

- Start in your boxing stance. Throw your lead hand straight from your chin while stepping out with your lead foot. Your elbow should go from your ribs straight up and out while your hand turns over to hit the target.
- Your hand should turn over your hand right before striking your target. Palm is facing down and your striking with your front two knuckles.
- Bring your hand back to your face, fast. Don't push your jab. Snap your jab.
- Keep your chin down and tucked in. While snapping jab out, your arm should go over your eye and tuck your chin down.

Different Jabs:

- Slip Jab: jab stays vertical.
- Body Jab: level change and snap jab while stepping forward towards target. Make sure to lean over and snap jab over and above eye to protect your head.

Note: jab is most important punch as it sets up all punches and can make your opponent react out of position.

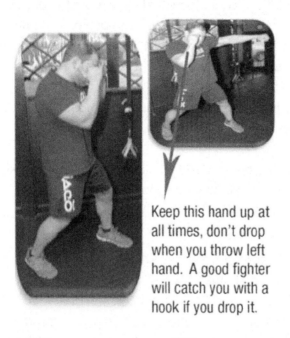

Keep this hand up at all times, don't drop when you throw left hand. A good fighter will catch you with a hook if you drop it.

Regular Jab **#1**   Slip Jab (vertical) **# 9**   Body Jab **# 5**

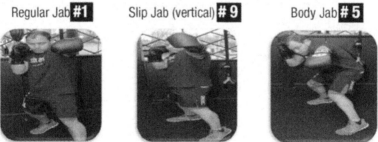

How to Throw a Power Hand #2:

- Start in your boxing stance. Throw your power hand from the ground up. Dig your right ball of foot into the ground as your pivot your heel out and towards your target. Make sure to sit back on the back heel even though it's 1-2 inches off the ground.

- Pivoting from the heel first should make your knee then hip pivot towards the target. Once your foot, knee and hip are turned then your elbow that's tucked into your side will rise to throw your punch along with the power hand shoulder.
- So, once your power fist hits the target. Your entire power side should be turned in this order. Foot > Knee > Hip> Shoulder to target.
- Your power hand should be thrown out while your chin tucks under your right shoulder. The right arm goes above eye level.
- Once the power hand hits the target, recoil quickly to be back into your boxing stance. Don't leave it out there.

Power Tips:

- Keep hands up always. Throw your power hand loose so it snaps. Don't muscle it.
- Sit back on your back foot when stationary. To throw a power hand when moving you'll have to step first with your lead foot then step up with your back foot while throwing the power hand.

Power Hand to The Body # 6: Same as the power hand to the head. Only difference is level changing before throwing the punch.

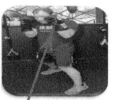

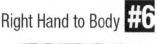
Right Hand to Body #6

Keep this hand up at all times, don't drop when you throw right hand. Remember, your opponent can throw his right hand, too.

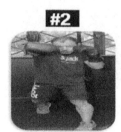

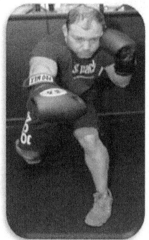

How to Throw Hooks:

Lead Hook (Head) #3:

- Start in your boxing stance. Practice feeling a hook by twisting your lead shoulder back to wind up and let a hook go out and around so as if you were punching around a tree. Your palm facing you or facing the ground, arm locked at 90 degrees and your elbow up at eye level.
- Pivot your heel out and turn your knee in to initiate the lead hook. Once your hook hits the target at the center point. Snap your fist back to your face.
- Once you get good at the hook, you should be able to throw it directly off your chin by just turning your arm over.
- Lead hook is best thrown after a power hand. One punch set up the other. Lead hooks are also thrown after a shovel punch to the body.

- Make sure to place 70% of your weight on your back foot by taking weight off your front ball of foot when throwing the lead hook. This will allow you to throw it with more speed.

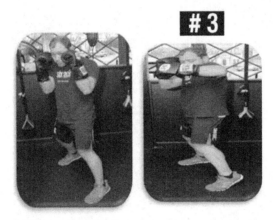

Back Hook (Head) #4:

- Start in your boxing stance. Initiate the back hook by turning your back heel out and around (pivot) on the ball of the foot. Make sure the weight is still back towards the heel to generate more power.
- Turn the heel, knee, hip and the back shoulder while throwing the back fist out and around with your palm always facing you.
- Again, the arm is 90 degrees and throw at eye level with your elbow up to protect your chin.

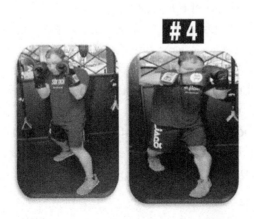

Lead Hook #7, Back Hook #8 (Body):

- Start in your boxing stance. Level Change down to the body. Lean slightly forward and throw similar to the head shots (same mechanics) but your throwing to the body.
- Snap your punches to the body.

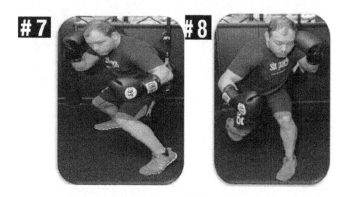

How to Throw an Upper Cut:

- Upper cuts are best thrown with power from your legs. Drive your palm out and up while turning your shoulder in that direction.
- Snap your upper cut up from your chin. Don't drop your hand below your neck line to throw the upper cut. Drop your body and throw off your face.
- Throw the upper cut from your chin not your chest.

Lead Upper Cut # 9:

Lean a bit to your lead side with a shift (slip) and turn up with power and speed. Snapping it up and back to your chin. Your hand comes off your chin when your turn your lead foot up.

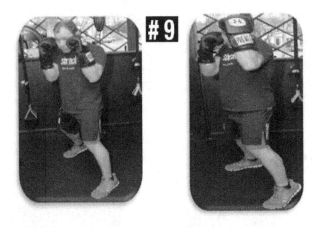

Back Upper Cut # 10:

Same principles as your hook with your lower body. Turn your heel, knee and hip towards direction of upper cut towards opponent's chin. Hand comes up and out towards your opponent's chin.

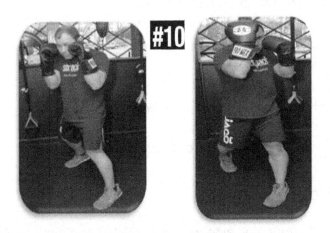

How to Throw a Shovel Punch:

- Shovel punches are mistaken for an upper cut. It's not. Shovel punch goes to the opponent's body.
- Level change and slip over to place pressure on the leg you'll be executing the shovel punch from either lead or back hand.
- Throw the upper cut from your chin not waist.

Lead Shovel Punch # 11:

- Lean a bit to your lead side with a shift (slip) and turn off with your lead foot (pivot heel). Throw your foot, knee and hip. Snap the punch up and in below the opponent's liver (below the rib cage). Fist should be at an angle with thumb up.
- Make sure your elbow is tucked into your side when throwing the punch in and up into your opponent.. Snapping it up and back to your chin. Your hand comes off your chin when your turn your lead foot up.

Back Shovel Punch # 12:

Same principles as your uppercut with your lower body. Turn your heel, knee and hip towards direction of upper cut towards opponent's chin. First, slip slightly over towards the side of your back foot and utilize your power to that side to throw the shovel punch towards the opponent's midsection.

Power Tips:

- Don't lean back when throwing the shovel punch. Place weight on your shovel punch side and lean slightly forward.
- Don't bring your elbow behind you to throw the punch.

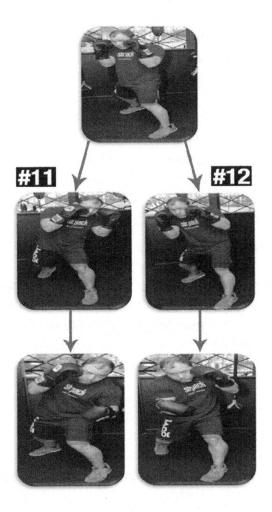

How to Throw an Overhand Punch (Knockout Punch) #14:

- Start in boxing position. Set up with a light jab. Step forward and slightly to the opposite side of your opponent with your lead foot.
- Simultaneously, bring your power hand of your chin and throw a looping punch up and over your opponent's jab hand. Punch in the trajectory of an arch.
- Important: when your step out with lead foot make sure to drop down by bending your front knee when throwing the

overhand punch. This will prevent your from leaning forward and falling on your face. Drop your weight down with the punch.

- Most of your weight will transfer to your front leg so make sure to bend that front knee with a level change.
- Your knuckles should be facing down towards the ground once your fist hits the target.
- Set up with a jab, fast straight power hand, lead hook etc..

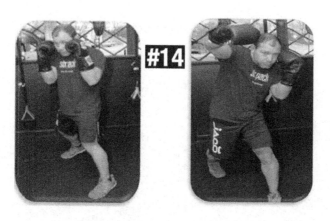

How to Move (Foot Work):

Stepping Forward:

- Start in boxing position. Step with your front foot 2-3 inches on the ball of the foot. Move by pressing off your back ball of the foot to step the same distance with your back foot.
- Make sure to initiate the forward movement with the lead foot. Step the front foot first then the back foot. Also, push off the back ball of the foot to straighten the back leg out to move forward. Move forward with force. DON'T slide the back foot on the ground. Pick it up to step.

Stepping should be like this, "Step Forward Foot, Step Back Foot, Step Forward Foot, Step Back Foot,…

Stepping Backward:

- Start in boxing position. Step with your back foot 2-3 inches on the ball of the foot. Move by pressing off your front ball of the foot to step the same distance with your front foot.
- Make sure to initiate the backward movement with the back foot. Also, push off the front foot to straighten the front leg to move backward with force. DON'T slide the front foot into position. Pick it up to step.

Stepping should be like this, "Step Back Foot, Step Front Foot, Step Back Foot, Step Front Foot…".

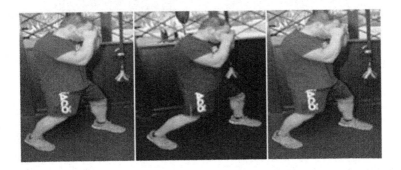

Stepping Side To Side:

Stepping Right (orthodox fighter example):

- Start in boxing position (orthodox stance with right foot back).
- Step with back foot 2-3 inches, then follow with the lead foot in the same distance.
- Don't drag your front foot

Stepping should be like this, "Step Back Foot right, Step Front Foot right, Step Back Foot right, Step Front Foot right…"

Stepping Left (orthodox fighter example):

- Start in boxing position (orthodox stance with right foot back).
- Step with front foot 2-3 inches, then follow with the back foot in the same distance.
- Don't drag your back foot

Stepping should be like this, "Step front foot left, Step back Foot left, Step front Foot left, Step Back Foot left…"

Stepping While Punching:

- Start in boxing position (orthodox stance with right foot back).
- Step forward with lead foot and jab at the same time.
- Now, step up with your back foot by picking it up and stick it into the ground equal to the same distance as the front foot moved. The key is to pick it up and stick it into the ground already turned (laces facing target, knee facing target and right hip facing the target). Notice below how the back hip rotates while the back foot steps forward.
- Hips shift left, right left, right and so on…

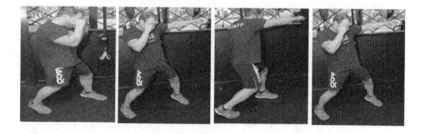

For Demo Video of all boxing exercises subscribe at
www.fitactions.com/builditworkoutvideos

Open Leg Shuffle:

- Start in squared stance with feet hip distance apart, slight squat, ball of feet, elbows tucked into side, gloves above your jaw and hands on your face.

- Keep this position at all time unless punching in which you'll switch from a square stance to your boxing stance to punch.
- Move to the right by moving your right foot to the right 3-4 inches and push off your left ball of foot to move right.
- Your left foot should move the same distance as your right.
- Repeat this movement around a circle (10 to 20 foot diameter).
- Circle 2x in the same direction. Once you get to the starting point, Front shuffle 6x each foot and then reverse the direction to do the same.
- Repeat both for 3 and/or 6 minutes

Variation:

- Every time you circle 1x, stop and get into your boxing stance and punch with one of the following combinations below:
- Punch #1,2 Punch #1,2,1 Punch #1,3,1 Punch #1,2,1,2,1
- Once you punch with speed and technique quickly shuffle in the other direction in your square stance for another 1x, stop and punch again in your boxing stance. Repeat the open leg shuffle with punches for 3 to 6 minutes.

NOTE: make sure to keep your hands up and elbows pulled in the entire time. Example below: step left foot and push off hard on the right foot into your starting position.

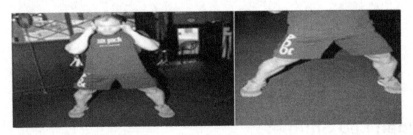

Boxing Level 1 (Foot Work)
Beginner: 3 min / Advanced: 3 min
Boxing Level 1 (Basic Punches)

BONUS WORKOUTS

BOXING WORKOUTS

Jump Rope	2 minutes
Foot Work (front to back, back to front)	2 minutes
Foot Work (right to left, left to right)	2 minutes
Foot Work (front to back, back to front) w 1,2,1	2 minutes
Foot Work (right to left, left to right) w/ 1,2,1	2 minutes
Open Leg Shuffle	2 minutes
Hop Right to Left, Left To Right 1,2	2 minutes
Shadow box 2,3,4,5 punch combinations w/ movment	2 minutes
Bag: 1,2 / 1,2,3 / 1,3 / 1,2,3,1	2 minutes
Bag: hooks (body, body, head, head)	2 minutes
Bag: Shovel (body, body)	2 minutes
Bag: hooks, shovel (hook: head,head, shove: body, body)	2 minutes
Jump Rope	2 minutes

Heavy Bag Tips:
- Change the tempo of your punches.
- Move around the bag.
- Vary up your combinations.
- Stay loose. Snap your punches out. Don't muscle them.
- Throw multiple combinations.
- Keep your range. Don't smother the bag unless throwing body punches (hooks, shovel punches).
- Shuffle around the bag, throw a combination and reverse direction. Don't stay in one spot.

- Always protect your hands and wrist with wraps.
- The leather heavy bag is best to purchase as they break in.

For heavy bag tips and workouts subscribe at
www. fitactions.com/builditworkoutvideos

DAY THREE/SIX			
BOXING WORKOUT			
Jump rope	2 x 3 minutes	3 x 3 minutes	4 x 3 minutes
Foot work	3 minutes	2 x 3 minutes	2 x 3 minutes
Foot work 1,2	1 minute	3 minutes	3 minutes
Cardio circuit	30 seconds	1 minute	2 x 1 minute
5 reps (push ups > mt climbers > down ups)			
Open leg shuffle	1 minute	2 minutes	3 minutes
Open leg shuffle punch	1 minutes	2 minutes	3 minutes
3 straight right with hop	30 seconds	1 minute	2 x 1 minute
Bag work: climb ladder	30 seconds	1 minute	2 x 1 minute
4-8 punch combination shadow	2 minutes	3 minutes	3 minutes
Bob and weave	1 minute	1 minute	1 minute
Bob and weave with 1,2,1,2	1 minute	1 minute	1 minute
Bag work: free style	3 minutes	2 x 3 minutes	3 x 3 minutes
Combo 2: jab-slip right-1,2,1,2 weave	3 minutes	2 x 3 minutes	3 x 3 minutes
Continuous upper cut	3 minutes	2 x 3 minutes	3 x 3 minutes
Continuous hook	3 minutes	2 x 3 minutes	3 x 3 minutes
Lateral jab drill:	3 minutes	2 x 3 minutes	3 x 3 minutes
1 right left 1,1 right left 1,1,1 right left	3 minutes	2 x 3 minutes	3 x 3 minutes
Jog	1 mile	2 miles	3 miles

Bag Work Combinations

1,2,3,1

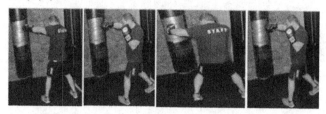

1,2,1

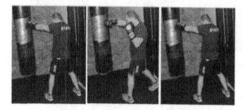

1,2,11,3,2

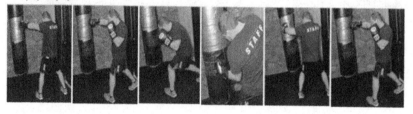

#1,11,14,1

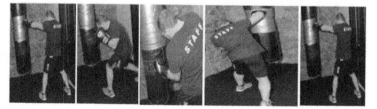

#1,2,1,14,1

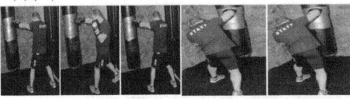

1,8,7,3,2,1

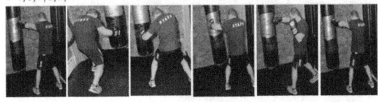

1,8,10,3,11,2,1

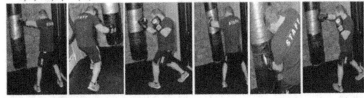

Other combinations to try:
1. # 1,1,2,2,3,9,1
2. # 1,1,2,11,2,10,2
3. #1,12,11,10,3,2,1
4. #1,5,10,3,2,1
5. # 1,13,14,11,3,2,1

FOOD BRANDS YOU MAY WANT TO TRY

NUTS AND BUTTERS

Natures-Way-Organic-Virgin-Coconut oil: great oil for any foods that you need oil.

Earth Balance butter Spread: great on ezekiel Toast or on baked potato. you'll skip the butter and definitely never eat margarine.

Spectrum Naturals Organic High Heat Peanut Oil: i like to add a tablespoon of this oil to veggies or pasta shells.

Spectrum Coconut Spray Oil: i use spectrums' oil sprays to oil pans for high heat. Trader Joes' and Whole foods has their own version which is as good.

Organic-Sea-Kelp-Delight-Seasoning: i've tried this on steak. not bad for super healthy mineral based seasoning. if you're looking to eat healthy than throw this in your cabinet.

Navitas Naturals Chia Seeds: great to get omega 3 into your diet. sprinkle on salads or add to smoothies.

Woodstock Farms Raw Almond Butter: great smooth taste. Best on Lunenburg brown rice cakes for breakfast or a quick hunger attack. Put sliced organic banana on top.

Teddie All Natural Peanut Butter: stir a tablespoon natural honey or grade a maple syrup into Teddies and you'll love it. So will your kids. I enjoy this on brown rice cakes.

Earth Balance Coconut and Peanut spread: if you're looking for a treat than try this peanut spread.

Justin's Nut Butter Natural Classic Almond Butter: great and handy lunch or on the go snack item. Try this with Bionaturae organic Wildberry fruit spread. classic PB & J but healthy.

Annie's Homegrown Organic Whole Wheat Shells & Cheddar: guys if you want a kick ass muscle meal than this is it. yup, mac and cheese but the non chicK Way: boil up some shells and put to side. step: 2, sauté lean natural buffalo meat, ground turkey or ground chicken in extra virgin olive oil. step 3: mix shells and meat together and take ½ packet along with some unsweetened almond milk and stir all together till smooth. step 4: add a 1 tsp Udo's choice oil 3 6 9 Blend or spectrums Peanut oil and mix again. Bang! you'll love it.

Lundberg Organic Brown Rice Cakes (Lightly Salted): hands down best brown rice cake on market. you need this in your cabinets and at work.

Bread Note: bread overall is not the best ab food but can be added for a balanced diet. Check out the breads below:

Mestemacher Sunflower Seed Bread: if you want a bread to throw some almond butter on than this is a good option. also, toast and try with your favorite soup.

Food For Life, Ezekiel 4:9 Bread, Original Sprouted, Organic: my bread of choice for last 15 plus years. great for everything needed for bread. i only eat this bread if i need too.

Udi's Gluten Free Breads: hands down the best commercial gluten free bread on the market.

Gillean's wheat and gluten free quiche pie crust: make your own quiche and impress your girl.

Engine 2: tortillas and hamburger rolls. Hamburger rolls are great toasted and topped with organic deli chicken or turkey. You can also toast them and place natural dairy free coconut cream cheese.

SOUPS

Note: soups are a great way to get veggies and protein in one meal. Portable and tasty if made right.

Amy's Organic Soups: my favorite are lentil, Tuscan bean rice and minestrone. you can actually get the multipack on amazon. amy's organic Variety Pack, Lentil (14.5-ounce) & minestrone (14.1-ounce) soup (Pack of 8)

Wolfgang Puck Organic Chicken with Egg Noodles Soup: good tasting canned soup for quick meal or snack.

Westbrae Natural Vegetarian Organic Soup Beans: not bad. i like to add cooked ground turkey or turkey bacon to this soup for extra protein and flavor. Parmesan cheese on top works well too.

Pacific Natural Foods: many soups to choose. The cashew ginger carrot is decent.

Trader Joe's Portuguese Fish Soup: taste like a chef made it in your own kitchen. Throw this on top of ½ cup brown rice and you've got a complete muscle meal.

Whole Foods prepared Chicken soup: tastiest and best soup around. Scoop with little broth and more chicken.

Pasta and Sauces:

Raos' Homemade Arrabbiata and marinara: mix this with organic pasta and veggies. spice gives a kick and you'll love the homemade taste. my "go to "sauce on gluten free brown rice pasta with ground lean chicken or turkey. Of course, fresh Romano on top (lots of it!).

Dinosaur barbeque sauces: wango tango and a few others will make you love barbeque sauce on just about anything.

Guy's Award Winning BBQ Sauce: if you're on a strict diet then I'd go with Guy's BBQ Sauce. Good taste.

Annies Marinades (teriyaki and smoky maple bbq): a great brand with great taste. The teriyaki will make chicken worth eating everyday. mix teriyaki with sautéed shitake mushrooms, onions, brown rice, cashews and chicken.

Annies Salad Dressings: try them all and go with 2-3 of your best ones.

Briannas Homestyle Salad Dressings: great with salad, chicken, beef and fish.

Newmans Own Salad Dressings: light italian and balsamic are good tasting.

Organic Apricot Preserves: Hands down the best thing to make protein taste gourmet. Whip 2-4 tsps. Into cooked ground turkey, cooked ground chicken, white tuna, organic plain yogurt, organic cottage cheese and/or with brown rice and raw nuts.

SNACKS (largest of list because this is where guys mess up)

Eden Organic Wild Berry Mix: I've added this to my snack mix. Little pricey compared to Trader Joe's Trail mix but a great brand. Try there pumpkin seeds, pistachios and dried cranberries.

Newman's Own Organics Spelt Pretzel: wheat free and a nuttier taste than most pretzels. i will have 2-3 of these for a quick crunch with my salad.

Go Raw Cookies: ginger snap, chocolate and original. Different than regular cookies but worth a try.

Justin's Organic Dark Chocolate Peanut Butter Cups: if you can eat just 1-2 (mini) per day on a maintenance plan you're ok. If you're addicted to sugar, refrain from eating them.

Perfect Bar: mini serving. Almond and peanut butter are great tasting and have little sugar. Found only in refrigerated section or on Amazon.

Tanka Bites, Spicy Pepper Blend: Extra protein.

Epic Bites, Spicy Pepper Blend: Extra protein.

Cold fusion sherbets: these are a tasty treat for that late night fix.

Whole Foods Cranberry Nut Mix: almonds, pumpkin seeds, dried cranberries and cashews.

Mary's Gone Crackers: best cracker on the market. All seeds. No flour. Original is the best tasting in my opinion.

Almond-licious ICE Supreme - Coconut Supreme:

Not a bad ice cream alternative. Give it a try. You may like it.

Terra Blue Chips: not a bad chip alternative. You can get them in 1 ounce bags. They are tasty so watch out.

Lundberg Organic Brown Rice Cakes (Lightly Salted): hands down best brown rice cake on market. you need this in your cabinets and at work. great with a tbsp. of all natural raw butter.

Natural Protein Powders and Supplements:

Orgain Organic Protein Powder: my go-to protein powder with frozen strawberries, scoop of amazing grass chocolate green superfood and tbsp. almond butter with unsweetened almond milk. Best tasting protein on the market. Not a body building protein. Best for the guys on the go who want to maintain muscle.

Vega Sport and Vega One protein: welcome to the new world of whole food proteins. Complete proteins for a real athlete. Yet, the aftertaste is a bit harsh and it is pricey but worth it if you can afford it. Not as good tasting as Orgain Organic Protein Powder.

Jarrow Formulas Whey Protein Chocolate: for chocolate you need to try this protein powder. It stirs so great and taste a little malty.

Now Foods Whey Protein Natural Unflavored: if you like whey protein than you'll enjoy now foods protein powders for their nutrition and taste.

Whole Foods Hemp or Whey Protein: similar to Trader Joe's store brand. Decent product for its price. Hemp protein is better than the whey protein for nutrition but you'll have to double up on the scoops for the much needed nutrition.

Amazing-Grass-Superfood: stir this with udo's oil blend in any smoothie. Little grassy but you'll get used to it.

Amazing-Grass-Amazing Meal Organic Chocolate Infusion Powder: great in your power smoothies or as a quick snack with unsweetened vanilla coconut or almond milk

PROTEIN AND DAIRY:

Crown Prince Natural Solid White or Light Tuna: texture is good and great with Trader Joe's spicy Peanut Vinaigrette

Pineland natural frozen beef patties: lean beef that's as natural as it gets for frozen patties. Keep these on hand in the freezer.

Applegate frozen organic beef burgers and turkey sausage: by far my favorite frozen beef and turkey sausages.

Wallaby Yogurt: best tasting regular yogurt. Tends to be little high in sugar but if you're not body building then don't worry about it.

Green Mountain Yogurt: check it out if you have it in your store. Best tasting.

Lisanatti Almond cheese Mozzarella and Cheddar style: dairy free cheeses that actually melt. Not the same as real dairy but not bad.

CEREAL

Barbaras shredded wheat: high in calories but packs a wallop for fiber. If you're gluten sensitive you better run from this product. Yet, best shredded wheat cereal on the market. Not bad for a treat or after heavy lifting with unsweetened almond milk and fresh organic blueberries.

Nature's Path Organic Flax Plus Multibran Cereal: if i were to eat cereal. This would be it. Great taste and high in fiber. If you're always hungry than take a bowl of this stuff.

Food For Life Ezekiel 4:9 Organic Sprouted Whole Grain Cereal: if you're going to eat cereal than eat this one. Give it a try with fresh blueberries and unsweetened almond milk. Great fiber and good after a long run.

Arrowheadmills Gluten Free steel cut oats: one of those gluten free foods that actually are good for you. Great Brand for oats, bran and other cereals.

Alpen all natural Muesli: one of those cereals that's more like a treat. Throw on some unsweetened almond milk and you'll have a filling snack.

Nature's Path Organic Instant Hot Oatmeal: as far as oatmeal goes natures Path is one of your best options. Plain steel cut oats are still the best for you. Yet, if you're maintaining a healthy lifestyle than give this oatmeal a try.

Wholefoods Cranberry Nut Mix: simply add unsweetened almond or coconut milk to a cup of the nut mix (cranberries, almonds, cashews and pumpkin seeds)

FROZEN FOODS:

PJ's Burritos: both the chicken and breakfast burritos are all natural and tasty. Put these in your freezer for a quick meal on the go.

Red's All natural Chicken Burrito: keep this chicken burrito in your freezer.

Evol Burritos: good tasting as far as frozen goes.

Glutino Gluten Free Pizza: if you like pizza once in a while and you eat gluten free then try this one.

Halal Cuisine: best frozen Indian food on the market. Chicken Biryani is the only one I eat. The rest of them are a little too high in fat.

Good Food Made Simple (breakfast burrito): chicken apple sausage is my favorite. I peel off ½ the wrap and throw it out. Microwave 2 min than toast for 2-3 minutes. Best tasting breakfast burrito I've found.

Amy's Bowls and Frozen Burritos: frozen dinners that are made of only the good stuff. Try them all and keep a few in the freezer for a quick meal to go.

Fresh Fields, Applegate Naturals and Plainville Farms Deli Meats: chicken, beef and turkey. Deli meats are not great for you but these are a great choice if you want a lean, natural cold cut sandwich. Only use with Ezekiel or Engine 2 Breads. Engine 2 hamburger rolls work great.

Cedars refrigerated salads (black bean/chickpea/ tabouleh): fresh, natural and girl approved for your dates. These are my go to little meals or side dishes when i'm in a rush.

AFTERWORD

Hey guys! Hope you learned something and you'll put this book into action. Again, if you read the beginning, I mentioned you won't get results by just reading it.

So, take action and kick your ass into shape.

Send any questions or comments to me personally, Doug bsstudio@comcast.net. I respond to all emails whether simple, positive, negative or complex.

If you're interested in working with me online at a higher level. Send me a request with the header, **"Interested in Your Online Training for Men."** My online training is unlike any training regimen in the fitness industry. My focus is for guys (entrepreneurs, executives, busy guys / age 30 – 60 years old/ gym, travel or home) who want to lose weight, build endurance, become stronger, learn boxing skills and live a high level of health and fitness.

Stay healthy !

Want to Work With Me Online for a Custom Program and/or Coaching?

Simply, send me an email (fitgy321@icloud.com) to learn more and set up a private coaching call.

-Doug

Made in the USA
Coppell, TX
25 January 2020

14991614R00154